Lies of the Magpie

Lies of the Magpie

Maleah Day Warner

JOIN the Magpie Discussion Group at:

www.facebook.com/groups/LiesoftheMagpie

Hosting a Book Club?

Download your FREE Book Club Discussion Questions at:
maleahwarner.com/book-club

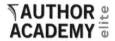

This is a work of creative nonfiction. The situations are portrayed to the best of the author's memory. While all of the events are true, certain incidents and characters have been composited for the sake of clarity and brevity. All names have been changed other than the names of the author and of Ms. Wickersham—the elementary school teacher—because with a name like Wickersham, no other pseudonym can suffice.

This book is dedicated to:

The Emily Effect
The Cook Family
The Dyches Family
Eric Dyches
Janean Rogers
Emily's Friends and Volunteers

In loving memory

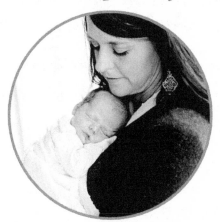

*A*t the start of 2016, I put the manuscript for this book away because I thought no one else would be interested in or would benefit from reading the story of my journey through postpartum depression.

Then I learned about the passing of our family friend, Emily Cook Dyches. Her family bravely shared her story and brought light, hope, healing, and change for so many.

I brushed off the manuscript and pressed forward.

This book is dedicated to Emily and to every mother who knows the darkness.

Maleah Day Warner

THE *emily* EFFECT

#Effect Change #End the Stigma
Visit: theemilyeffect.org

We live by the grace of story.
Another woman's story saved me.
I arrived on her doorstep, uninvited, after midnight.

Porcelain women carry the burden of humanity.
We crack under the weight,
Other women come—elves in the night—
And use stories as glue to join us together.

My story merits telling.
It is true.
And it is mine.

mw

Contents

BOOK THREE: CHANGE

PROLOGUE

The Magpie Rhyme

One for sorrow,
Two for mirth,
Three for a funeral
And four for birth
Five for silver
Six for gold,
Seven for a secret,
Never to be told.
Eight for a wish,
Nine for a kiss,
Ten for a bird,
You must not miss

Traditional Children's Nursery Rhyme

Ambition

FROM A YOUNG age I had dreams of growing up to be wildly successful.

I also had buck teeth, and it's difficult to say which was more pointed, my ambition or my profile.

I remember the day my fourth-grade teacher, Ms. Wickersham, asked me The Big Question: "What do you want to be when you grow up?"

I remember exactly.

It was the day we ran from the magpies.

After teaching a lesson on long division, Ms. Wickersham traded her dress pumps for a pair of sturdy white sneakers to walk laps around the school grounds during morning recess. As usual, I forfeited playing with kids my own age in favor of adult interaction. I was a straggly thing, as knotted and lanky as an old fence post with stringy brown hair that hung in clumps of snarls. Ms. Wickersham's hair was a marvel to me. She stood at the chalkboard writing multiplication tables, her short glossy waves shaped into stiff points with frosted tips, like the multiple peaks of white meringue on a lemon pie. Her hair never moved, even when an autumn breeze through the open window blew papers from her desk.

Ms. Wickersham had come all the way from Pennsylvania to teach elementary school in this one-horse town nestled in the castle rock formations of eastern Utah. An ardent Pittsburgh Steelers fan, she decorated our classroom with football pendants and drank steaming coffee from a black and gold mug. When the Steelers lost, we tormented Ms. Wickersham to hysterics until she reverted to speaking with her thick East Coast accent, which launched the class into stomach-grabbing fits of laughter. Her language was so different from the country-western drawled in our coal mining county. Unlike the rest of our teachers, we never saw Ms. Wickersham in church on Sundays. She might have been the first non-Mormon I'd ever met.

Catching up to Ms. Wickersham's brisk pace, I sidled up and became her chatty walking partner. By age nine I had well-earned the nickname "motor mouth" due to a talkative streak that provoked my brothers to chase me down and seal duct tape over my mouth when they grew tired of listening to me ramble on in paragraphs without taking a breath. For years I believed the silver adhesive was called "duck" tape because—in theory—you could wrap it around a duck's bill to stop the incessant quacking.

Also by age nine, I had noticed that when grown-ups found themselves with the awkward necessity of making conversation with a child, they defaulted to the topic of what you want to be when you grow up. When Ms. Wickersham asked me The Big Question, I was prepared with a long-winded answer. I took a big breath, poised to impress another grown-up with my lengthy list of aspirations.

"I want to be a lot of things," I said, brimming with self-confidence and not a trace of arrogance, the way only children can. "I want to be a singer and a dancer." I gave her an unsolicited performance there on the sidewalk. She applauded politely. "I want to be a nurse, a writer, a teacher, an astronaut"—I had fantasies of being the first woman in outer space—"a fire fighter, a writer..." Usually, my list ended with writer, but I'd just discovered the book *A Wrinkle in Time* by Madeline L'Engle and had found my newest role model. I had no interest in being Meg, the main girl character. Mrs. Murry, the scientist/mother with a chemistry lab built off her kitchen, was far more appealing. I stopped walking and planted both feet. "And I want to be a scientist."

Ms. Wickersham also stopped walking. She looked at me standing there big as life in my home-sewn polyester jumpsuit, seventy pounds of undiluted aspiration. "You want to be all those things?" She raised her painted eyebrows to the level of her tinted hair.

I looked up at her with all the intensity my brown eyes could muster. "Yes, I want to do all those things. I have a lot of interests."

"Don't you want to be a mother?" Ms. Wickersham asked.

This was 1983. My childhood was sandwiched between the 1980s feminist movement and my conservative religious upbringing. I formed my words carefully in order to please any traditional housewives or glass ceiling-breakers who might be eavesdropping on this nine-year-old's intentions.

"Yes, of course I'll be a mother."

"How many brothers and sisters do you have?" Ms. Wickersham asked, resuming our walk.

"Five brothers and two sisters. There are eight kids in my family," I answered.

Ms. Wickersham clicked her tongue. "Your mother is *a-maz-ing*."

For the first time during the walk, I was quiet. What did my mom do that was *a-maz-ing*? She wore an apron most of the day and spent a lot of time in the kitchen. When my five brothers and our dog got too shaggy, she tied them to a chair and gave them haircuts. She milked the cow if Dad was out of town and led the music in church. She talked on the phone while baking six loaves of bread a week and chocolate chip cookies on Saturdays. Everything I wore she had created in her sewing room, from frilly Easter dresses to my lace-trimmed underpants. But I didn't know what Ms. Wickersham meant because my mom didn't do anything special outside of being a mom. In my mind, being a mother didn't make a woman *a-maz-ing*.

"I plan to have six or seven kids," I affirmed to Ms. Wickersham, "but I won't just be a mom. I want to do all those other things, too." I pictured myself wearing a white lab coat over my apron—or was it an apron over my white lab coat?—exactly like Mrs. Murry.

"That is very ambitious," Ms. Wickersham said.

"Oh, I have a lot of ambition," I assured her.

Walking under a willow tree in a far corner of the school property, I felt a wet splatter and raised my arm to see white goop laced with brown stripes dripping down my elbow. Ms. Wickersham took a tissue from her pocket and wiped the mess while I scanned the tree for the bird who had pooped on me. A blur of black and white swooped low, brushing the top of Ms. Wickersham's head. She took off her sun hat and waved it. "Shoo. Fly away bird."

The bird glided up and landed on the chain link fence. A similar bird flew out from the tree and sat on the fence next to the first. Their eyes were dark and glossy, like the favorite marbles in my collection. They pivoted their heads with sharp movements, looking wildly around, seeming to gather what news they could about this place. A breeze whooshed by and I turned to see three more black and white creatures landing on the grass behind us.

"Let's keep walking." Ms. Wickersham nudged my shoulder. "These birds make me nervous."

"Why?" I asked.

"Oh, it's a silly superstition. How many magpies you see tells if you will have bad or good luck."

There were magpies on our farm, but I never knew they meant good or bad luck. My dad called them "pesky scavengers." Nothing scared them. They taunted our farm dog, working him into running dizzy circles while they stole the very food out of his dog pan during the distraction. Then, for fun, they helped themselves to dessert from the cat's bowl. Before daily chores, my dad would remind us, "Don't put too much food in the pets' dishes. I'm going to spend my whole living feeding those thieving birds."

Behind us a sharp chirping erupted. We turned around to see a row of magpies lined up neatly like tin soldiers. The birds squawked, hopping and cocking their heads, exchanging gossip and closing in on us. "Oh...OH!" Ms. Wickersham hopped back as a bird swooped up and made a grab for her shiny earring. "Down, bird. Shoo!" Ms. Wickersham danced in a circle, flapping her hat at the air. A different bird darted up and bit the silver buckle on my belt. We were caught in a flurry of feathers. Ms. Wickersham removed her silver bracelet and held it out for the birds to see. "Here, birdies. Look." She wiggled the bracelet to reflect the sun's light. Once the birds were watching, Ms. Wickersham tossed the bracelet under the willow tree and grabbed my hand. "Run!"

We ran down the hill and didn't stop until we arrived at the playground where the squeals of school children replaced the magpie's squawking. Ms. Wickersham bent over, catching her breath. I giggled seeing the terror on her face. "Why did you give them your bracelet?" I wondered why she would part with such a beautiful treasure.

"Magpies love anything shiny that sparkles. It was worth one bracelet to save our lives, don't you think?" She knelt down in front of me and reached behind her head to unclasp her necklace. It had a ruby gem shaped like a heart that matched her bracelet.

Ms. Wickersham linked the chain around my neck. She massaged her fingers and pulled off a loose Lee Press On Nail. "I've lost a bracelet and a fingernail to those magpies"—she was still catching her breath—"I want you to keep the necklace safe where it won't get lost."

My eyes grew huge and my hands circled the ruby heart as if it were a crystal ball with a message I desperately needed to understand.

"Make a wish and kiss the gem and it will bring you the greatest desires of your heart."

My eyes sparkled and I smiled widely.

Ms. Wickersham winked. "Thank you for telling me about your dreams, Maleah. You are a special girl. I can't wait to see what great things you will grow up and do in the world."

I hugged Ms. Wickersham tightly around the neck, breathing in her scent of perfume and coffee. With closed eyes, I kissed the gemstone and made my silent wish.

I wish to grow up to be the most amazing woman in the world.

Nothing about my gangly appearance or small-town roots deterred me in the least. I was headed for fame and fortune. It seemed that

Destiny herself had kissed my cheek, marking me for glory with her lipstick.

AFTER RECESS, A new student was sitting at my table. She looked unattached and hungry for an ally. She was nearly as boney as me, practically a stick figure. Scooting my chair close to hers, I asked if she could keep a secret. Pulling the chain with the ruby gem from under my shirt, I told her the story of Ms. Wickersham and the special necklace. She promised to keep my secret. She told me her name was Laiah, pronounced with a long *i* sound, like *LI*-ah that rhymes with papaya. Her name, like mine, sounded Hawaiian, though neither of us were from Hawaii. I whispered that my name was Maleah, pronounced with a long *e* sound, like Ma-*LEE*-ah that rhymes with Maria. We shared a desk and a pencil box and became inseparable companions. For years we were *Maleah Maria* and *Laiah Papaya*. I felt more complete the day she joined me on my chair than I ever had. There was something about her that I needed. Every day after school, under my dad's camper shell in our back yard, Laiah played Meg to my Mrs. Murry. "Add some salt to the stew, will you, Meg?" I'd say, adjusting the safety goggles over my eyes, "and don't get mixed up with the boric acid this time, please." Laiah would do anything I said. I had met my match.

LOOKING BACK NOW, I have to wonder if it was just me, or did every little girl grow up believing she was special? Did other girls leave their hometowns lassoing dreams the size of a Texas sky, with a rope of ambition equal to the span of those dreams? I never thought of it at the time, but today if I could go back to that moment with Ms. Wickersham, the ruby necklace, and The Big Question, I would stop, look straight in her eyes and ask, "What do you think happens, Ms. Wickersham, when ambitious girls grow up to be *mothers?*"

Book One

The Road to Tucson

CHAPTER 1

The Argument

Thursday 1:00 p.m.

THE ROAD AHEAD is long and isolated, winding through a vast panorama of nothingness. I lean into the steering wheel and scan the horizon. *Nothing.* The arid desert spans in all directions and it seems I'm the only human within miles of lonely saguaro cacti.

"Go faster!" I urge the car forward, pressing the gas pedal to the floor, but still the barren scenery passes too slowly. I feel more like a pioneer driving a rickety wagon while whipping the back of an ornery mule than a modern woman speeding across Arizona at ninety miles per hour in her husband's gold Ford Taurus. The June sun glares through the windshield turning the car into a furnace, even though the air conditioner is blowing full power in a futile effort to keep me, and my enlarged belly, from overheating.

Maybe I should have stayed home.

Not one vehicle has passed me in thirty minutes, and the isolation of this road has me worried that I'm not on I-10. There should be more traffic on a major interstate. Did I take the wrong exit? Thinking back to the tangle of belt loops and bridges that make up the Phoenix metro system, I'm questioning if I followed the right spaghetti noodle off the plate. At one point I-10 was pointed due east, now it seems I'm going south. At least, I *think* I'm headed south. I have the geographic sense of a dodo bird in a cyclone.

I'm supposed to be driving to Tucson to attend the Arizona State Music Teachers annual convention, but this bleak, unchanging landscape has me so turned around until I can't discern north from south or east from west. My husband, Aaron, had spewed off hasty directions as I ran out the door at noon, but I should have taken the time to print the route from MapQuest instead of cleaning the bathrooms. For all I know, I may not be driving toward Tucson at all. I might be headed into the forsaken Black Canyons of New Mexico.

For a moment I consider calling to ask Aaron for help figuring out where I am. He jokes that I need directions to find my own house. Before I can type his number, a tightening pinch begins in my back and wraps to the front. The contraction pulls and twists.

"Ouch!" I brace myself with gritted teeth and fight against the pain, my spine arching in opposition. A howling siren sound emerges from my throat, starting low then rising high and falling again to cover several octaves. Any vocal coach would be impressed. Little by little, the tension eases. *Breathe*, I remind myself, but another contraction is climaxing before the first recedes, followed by yet another. Minutes click past on the clock. Three contractions in a row without a break. If my water breaks here in Aaron's car, I'll never be able to clean away the stench of amniotic fluid. Aaron's nose can track a lost sippy cup the moment the milk turns sour.

The person I need to talk me through this is Laiah. She has been my confidante for so long, I can hardly boil water without her input. Instead of dialing Aaron, I call on Laiah for help. "The contractions are getting harder and I don't know what road I'm on!" I tell her. "Should I call Aaron or turn around and go back home?"

Laiah's voice rings loud and clear. "You can do this," she coaches. "Hang in there. This happens to you every pregnancy. These contractions will go away after a while."

Laiah is right. This is my fourth baby and for whatever unknown reason, my uterus contracts more than a team of corporate lawyers.

The hardest part of my pregnancies is knowing the right time to go to the hospital.

"You asked me to remind you that this is exactly what happened with your last pregnancy. Well, this is me reminding. You do not want a repeat of what happened when Tanner was born."

I cringe at the memory of my third delivery two years ago. I can't allow myself to repeat the same mistakes I made with Tanner's birth. "But these contractions feel so real," I plead to Laiah.

"You can stay home and miss the conference, but I know you and you'll regret it," Laiah points out. "You'll waste the weekend counting contractions and second-guessing if you should go to the hospital. You will drive yourself and Aaron crazy. You know he hates it when you're indecisive. Besides, you can't call Aaron. Not after what happened last night."

———⦿⦿⦿———

AARON DIDN'T WANT me to leave. Last night while I packed my suitcase, Aaron paced the bedroom.

"Are you seriously planning to leave this close to your due date?"

"I've hardly had any contractions today. I'll be fine."

Aaron stood on the opposite side of the bed. "You had a ton of contractions on Tuesday, remember? You almost went to the hospital. How many weeks along are you?"

"Thirty-seven." I lowered my head and my voice with the comment. A typical pregnancy lasts forty weeks. Technically, I'm at thirty-seven and one-half weeks, but I didn't mention the one-half to Aaron.

"Weren't Danny, Kate, and Tanner *all* born at thirty-seven weeks?" Aaron pressed.

I nodded slightly. Kate was born at thirty-six weeks, but I didn't see fit to remind Aaron of that fact, either.

"Who are you driving with?"

I'd signed up for the conference thinking I would carpool with other piano teachers. That was how I discovered I'm the only registered piano teacher west of Glendale.

"You're driving alone?" Aaron shouted.

"It's not that far. I'll be fine."

"Tucson is a four-hour drive."

Four hours? I didn't realize Tucson was so far away. Other than mailing in the registration check, I hadn't done anything to prepare for this conference. Still, I continued folding clothes and adding them to the case. "This training is only once a year. If I don't go this weekend, I have to wait for next summer."

Aaron stormed over and closed the suitcase lid, nearly smashing my fingers and forcing me to look at him. "Can you please explain how this is a good idea, to drive four hours in a car by yourself when every other baby has been born at thirty-seven weeks? Based on your track record, the baby is coming this weekend." Aaron flung his arms.

"Piano is important to me." The words came out quietly and I wasn't sure he heard me.

When I was fourteen, I won first place in my local Farm Bureau Talent Find. The emcee pinned a blue ribbon on my dress—one of those ruffled county fair-style ribbons, the same ones they tape to the sweepstakes-winning bottle of peach preserves or tie around the horn of the grand champion bull. Then he shook my hand while handing me a trophy and a $100 savings bond. The audience applauded.

The town reporter asked everyone to move aside while he snapped photos of me with my prizes and asked how to spell my name.

"M-a-l-e-a-h." I tilted my head and smiled for the camera.

Then one of the judges pulled me away from my circle of congratulators. "It wasn't even a competition tonight," he said, still holding my elbow and whispering, "the second-place winner didn't touch the bottom of your shoes."

I stared at this stranger who had come from another town to judge the competition. Why was he going out of his way to tell me this?

"You have a special touch for Chopin. The audience was in the palm of your hand. No one breathed until you played the very last note."

My heart pounded.

"You are the most impressive young woman I have ever met. I hope you'll never stop playing. You were absolutely dazzling." He extended his hand and I hoped he wouldn't notice the sweat on my palm as he shook my hand with gusto. "Congratulations on tonight, you deserved it." Then he walked out of the building.

"Who was that?" my mother asked, coming over and straightening the ribbon on my dress.

"One of the judges," I said.

"What did he say?"

"He liked my performance."

The next Tuesday morning Laiah looked over my shoulder at the picture of me on the front page of the newspaper. "You look so pretty," she said. The dress I'd worn made my fourteen-year-old figure look more curvy than usual. On that morning, like every other Tuesday morning, farmers and miners and teachers were picking up their newspapers and they were all looking at *me*, the talent winner of the county. I could not stop smiling.

But standing across the bed, Aaron was not smiling. "Hmm? Tell me how you think driving alone is a good idea!" He bounced his leg waiting for my answer.

I took a deep breath, gearing up to—once again—try to explain what I desperately wanted Aaron to understand. "The only reason Kate and Tanner were born at thirty-seven weeks is because I went to the hospital *too* early. Any hospital will admit a woman who is thirty-seven weeks and contracting. Both times the doctor insisted on giving me Pitocin or breaking my water to speed up labor. Ever since Tanner's birth, I've wondered how far I can make it if I don't panic and go to the hospital too soon."

Aaron looked at me as if I had bird seed for brains. He couldn't understand why going full-term was important to me. Despite being born three weeks early, each of our babies have been healthy with fully developed lungs and hungry tummies—no premature birth complications, no oxygen machines, no feeding tubes, no extended hospital stays. As far as Aaron was concerned, going to the hospital at thirty-seven weeks and getting a shot of Pitocin was as sensible a way to have a baby as hooking up jumper cables to start a car battery. But it wasn't for me. If this was our last baby, I wouldn't get another chance to see if I could carry a pregnancy a full forty weeks.

I looked in Aaron's eyes hoping to see a glint of the adoration he used to have for me. I wanted him to take me in his arms and say, "You are so strong. So brave. I'm lucky to be married to you."

Instead of marveling at my moxie, Aaron got even more fired up. "If your water breaks, I will never make it to Tucson in time."

Why does he still doubt me? Haven't I worked hard enough these past ten months to prove he didn't get a lemon when he married me? I have said yes to everything. Yes to teaching early-morning Bible study. Yes to starting a business. Yes to traveling. Yes to hosting. Even my ovaries and uterus had jumped on *the Year of Saying Yes* bandwagon.

The only way I can think to impress Aaron is to perform better on this delivery than I did on my previous three births. I have to be strong. "My water won't break."

Aaron stopped the leg bouncing. He held his arms out in front as if he were pleading. Only after several seconds of silence did he speak, almost in a whisper. "Stay home." His voice was a blanket of exasperation. "You don't have to go to the hospital this weekend, but don't go to Tucson either."

What I couldn't say to Aaron was that if I stayed home, I was afraid I wouldn't have the willpower to keep myself out of the hospital.

More seconds of silence ticked away before I answered. "Nothing is going to happen." I spoke the words to the clothes in my suitcase, not looking at Aaron. "Besides, I've already paid the $350 registration fee. It's nonrefundable."

Without looking up, I could feel Aaron stare at me in disbelief, but he shouldn't have been surprised. He had been married to me long enough to know that if it came down to losing money or making a sage decision, I would chase after the money every time.

Aaron dropped his hands. "No one can make you do anything you don't want to do." He expelled a sigh of surrender.

I had won.

Aaron left the room with a grunt of frustration.

My arms caught the weight of my body as I fell forward, instantly feeling the regret of pushing back so hard. I'd gotten so caught up in the fight, I'd forgotten the cost of winning. Tomorrow I would be driving to the conference alone. *What if my water did break in Tucson?*

Aaron's heavy footsteps sounded down the hall followed by the heavy thud of the office door closing. There was a time, years ago, when everything about me made Aaron ooze with love and admiration. Now, it seems I only fill him with agitation.

CHAPTER 2

Admiration

MY FAST-PACED WALK around campus is what Aaron remembers most about me from college. He played tennis at the courts across from my off-campus housing. For weeks he watched me leave my apartment, hurry across the road, rush past the tennis courts, shortcut across the grass, and disappear into the humanities building. His tennis partner noticed him staring and said, "Don't waste your time. That is Maleah Day. She's the academic vice president. She walks that fast everywhere she goes. Ten bucks says you can't get her to stop to talk to you."

It was my sophomore year. I was ten years older than the straggly nine-year-old girl from Ms. Wickersham's fourth grade class. My bean-pole figure had filled out in a few key places. Two years of orthodontic work and contact lenses had tamed my profile, but my ambition—if possible—was still as potent. I declared a political science major and carried an application for the Peace Corps in my backpack. My scholarship covered full tuition and fees for unlimited credit hours, so in addition to social sciences, I loaded my transcript with biochemistry, anatomy, and microbiology in case I changed my mind about foreign diplomacy and decided on medical school. By the time Aaron first spied me speed-walking past the tennis courts, I already had one year of college life under my belt. I was a proficient calendar-juggler, balancing twenty credit hours and every extracurricular activity that would either look good on my resume or provide free dinner. For me, college was an all-you-can-eat buffet and I planned to devour my money's worth.

Aaron didn't have a clue what he was getting into the day he rested his tennis racquet on his shoulder, leaned casually against the chain link fence, and called out, "Hey there beautiful girl!" as I hurried to yet another important appointment.

Hearing a voice, I glanced up, but didn't slow down. Boys didn't often talk to me. It wasn't that I was unattractive, more like inaccessible. I had graduated from high school as a card-carrying member of the virgin lip club, well—the virgin everything club. Laiah assured me, "One day your assertiveness and 4.0 GPA will attract boys instead of intimidate them." In the meantime, I accumulated a dowry of personal accomplishments, trusting that when I was ready to consider marriage, I would be an enticing catch. One day I would find the boy who would take a risk to get to know me, who would be brave enough to love me.

Aaron jogged along the fence to keep up with me. "Hey there. What's up? What's the rush?" I recognized his face from a picture in the student council office. He was campaigning for a seat in the Freshman Senate, an office elected by popular vote. My position as the academic vice president had been faculty appointed. He put his tennis racquet in his left hand and offered me his sweaty right palm. "I'm Aaron Warner." His flirty smile made me both flattered and flustered.

"Oh. Hi. I'm Maleah Day." I looked apologetically at his still-extended hand. "Sorry, my hands are full." I nodded down to the stack of books balanced beneath my chin.

He tossed his racquet onto the grass and reached out for the books. "Here, let me take those."

The sound of his voice sent an electric current through me. I gripped the books to my chest. It could not be healthy to feel so instantly attracted. What would Laiah say? We'd agreed on multiple occasions not to let silly boys distract us. She scoffed at girls who wasted college studying men rather than books. "You don't want to be the girl who has no ambition beyond being a man's wife." While marriage and family were on my to-do list, there were so many things I wanted to do first, like join the Air Force and work in Washington D.C., but those things *after* eighteen months of volunteer missionary service.

"No, it's okay. I've got them." I pulled the books closer. "I'm presenting to the Faculty Academic Council on boosting the school's transfer credit rating, but all the course catalogues I'd highlighted were at my apartment, so I had to run back to get them and now I'm almost late." The words spilled onto the sidewalk where my racing feet tripped over them as I made a sharp left turn and started to run, my dress pumps clicking loudly on the sidewalk. "Sorry I can't stay and chat. I have to hurry, or I'll never make it."

"Will you be at the campaign rally this Friday?" Aaron called as the humanities building door closed behind me. "Maybe I'll see you there?" he questioned the empty space where I'd just been. He didn't know about my celibacy record or how I was terrified that dating would thwart my run for success. He didn't know I'd been awake since 5:30 a.m., cramming in hours of classes, homework, and meetings. All he knew was there was a brown-haired, brown-eyed girl who had nearly given him the brushoff, and he felt up to the challenge.

———⟨∅∅∅⟩———

THE NEXT FRIDAY night, I did go to the campaign rally—not to socialize, but to fulfill my obligations as a student body officer. It was late September and college students gathered in a canyon east of campus. On such a beautiful evening, I was relieved to have a resume-worthy excuse to be outdoors instead of feeling guilty about not studying. The leaves of the scrub oak burned brilliant red and the aspen trees transformed their top hats from green to yellow. The sound of a mountain breeze rustling through these colored leaves is why the trees are called "quaking" aspens.

I stood in the back of the crowd, my hands wrapped around a Styrofoam cup of hot chocolate and watched Aaron deliver a confident "Why You Should Vote for Me" speech. He stood on a platform set up next to the bonfire. Nobody could hear the other speeches above the crackle of the fire and the buzz of socializing, but when Aaron stood on the platform to speak, everybody could hear him and everybody listened. He exuded an air of trustworthy confidence and spontaneous playfulness. When he stood in front, the crowd seemed to say, "Yes, we will follow him because he will take us where we want to go and we will have fun along the way."

The fire compounded the natural spark that already resided in his eyes. I liked the contours of his face—the distinct jawline and cheekbones, but especially his eyes accented by long, dark lashes, and wavy brown hair. He didn't seem fazed by anything. He certainly wasn't intimidated tonight, not by this noisy crowd and not by being in the spotlight. I tried to decide if he knew how attractive he was.

"Are you swooning?" From out of nowhere, Laiah appeared. "There's no doubt he's charismatic, and evidently you're not the only girl here to be seduced by his charm." Laiah drew my attention away from Aaron to the rows of girls around me, giggling as they watched his speech.

"Oh brother." I rolled my eyes, embarrassed for myself. I had already vowed, on multiple occasions, that I would never stoop to primping, flirting, tilting my chin, or high-pitched giggling—all to win a little masculine attention. I nodded. It was time to leave. I had squandered enough of my time at this campus activity. "I'm going home to work on my paper."

Laiah stayed close as we walked away. "A guy like that would mean nothing but distraction and trouble for you," she whispered in my ear, but when she wasn't watching, I turned my head to sneak one more glance. Aaron had finished speaking and was surrounded by a gaggle of girls vying for his attention. Not in the least befuddled by the circus of flirtatiousness, he had them leaping through hoops in a circle around him. From the center of the panoply, Aaron looked out, his eyes searching. The exhibition seemed to move in slow motion until his eyes found me and he captured my gaze. I didn't look away. How did he know I was here? Despite the feminine festivity all around him, his eyes made me feel that I was the only girl that mattered.

—◦◦◦—

Thursday 1:15 p.m.

I WASN'T HAVING contractions before I left home, but I may have overexerted in the rush to stock up with groceries and mop the tile floor. I couldn't leave Aaron wrestling our three kids for the weekend in a messy house with no food and not feel guilty. The past year has been grueling. Once this baby comes, Aaron will resign from his nine-to-five job and come home to help me with the printing business we started. For six months my swollen feet have been pounding the pavement, carrying me from business to business soliciting advertisers for our magazine in hopes to grow our sales revenue faster than my circumference. The thought of two relaxing nights in a hotel room by myself is divine, and now these contractions are throwing a wrench in my chance for some R&R.

Another tightening begins low in my abdomen and winds like a pair of boa constrictors, snaking their way up around my torso in opposite directions and compressing with all their might. I grimace and squint my eyes, leaving open a narrow slit of vision, just enough to see the road speeding beneath my tires. Meanwhile, Laiah's voice is on loud speaker. She likes to talk and I need her gift of distraction if I'm going to make it through this drive. Laiah chatters away while I hold the steering wheel in a death grip that drains the blood from my knuckles. At last the contraction lets go, leaving me wrung out like a wet dishrag.

Aaron doesn't seem to appreciate what I go through to have these babies. It's been a long time since I've done anything that really impressed him. "Remember when Aaron used to think I was so amazing?" I ask Laiah.

"Yes. In student council meeting, he used to stare at you across the room like you were the most incredible woman in the universe. He thought you were perfect."

My mind floods with memories from that year in college, when I was everything that Aaron had ever hoped to find in a woman.

———◈———

AARON WON THE election. As a freshman senator he moved into a desk across from mine in the student government office. We saw each other nearly every day at meetings, during leadership class, and he sat behind me in calculus. At one meeting, Cory, the student body president, stood up to conduct. "I guess we should start by announcing that our debate team took first place over the weekend and qualified for nationals. Coach Warbler told me that Maleah here led the team and broke a tournament record by trophying in four events." Cory spoke with school pride.

I caught Aaron looking at me. A tingle went down my spine.

After the meeting I heaved my pack of books onto my back and made a beeline for the door. Aaron caught my arm before I could exit. "Congrats on the debate win. I wondered why you weren't at the dance Friday. I looked for you."

He looked for me? I imagined dancing with Aaron and my legs turned to jelly. "Yeah, we left Thursday and didn't get back until"—I looked at my watch—"about three hours ago. We drove all night. How was the dance?" I wondered who he had danced with. If I had been there, would he have asked me to dance?

"It was fun, but it would have been better if you had been there."

My stomach fluttered. This boy was not good for me. "I haven't seen you in calculus for a while," I said, changing the subject.

"That's because I haven't gone to calculus for a while." Aaron pulled me away from the doorway, letting the other council members exit and committing me to a longer conversation. There were vibrations in my skin where his hand touched my wrist. "I dropped that class," he said. "I couldn't figure out K Pi from cow pie, it was all a bunch of crap to me." His smile filled the room and I couldn't help laughing.

"What do you know about cow pies?" I asked.

"I know cow pies," he said. "I worked for a dairy farm in high school. I've thrown a few toxic Frisbees in my day."

I hadn't pegged him as a farming sort of fellow. I came from generations of cattle, sheep, and dairy farmers—a fact I didn't openly share. Aaron laughed and I watched his eyes dance. His green eyes. I had a weakness for green eyes.

"Time to go," Laiah mouthed, tapping her watch.

"I've gotta run or I'll be late for ballet." I ducked under the arm he had stretched out between the door and me. As I hurried down the hallway, I wanted to turn around to see Aaron's face again. Instead, I absorbed the feeling of his eyes watching me rush away.

CHAPTER 3

Love & Marriage

LAIAH WAS THE first to see the flyer advertising the homecoming royalty pageant. "You should enter." She ripped the flyer from its tack and handed it to me. "The winner gets a cash scholarship and a new computer." I filled out the pageant application, submitted a photo, and borrowed a dress.

The night of the pageant I was pacing backstage waiting for my turn in the talent competition when I heard a voice call to me. "Hey stranger." Aaron walked toward me dressed in a sleek, black tuxedo, a ginormous grin covering his face.

"Well, you clean up pretty well," I said, taking in his aura. His hair was slicked with gel. He straightened his bow tie and winked at me, looking like a *GQ* model. I was already nervous, wringing my hands and pulling at my numb fingers. His presence filled me with electricity and I wobbled unevenly in my high-heeled shoes, fighting to stay balanced. The air in the dark backstage was frigid, but suddenly I felt an odd mix of hot and cold, as if my entire body had been placed in a furnace, except my arms, which were in a freezer. I rubbed my shoulders, my wrists, my palms together and blew into them as if I were standing outside in a snowstorm. "What are you doing here?" I asked Aaron, trying to sound completely calm and in control.

"Madame Pageant Director asked the senators to be your escorts this evening," he spoke with an exaggerated, sophisticated accent. "I just wanted to tell you good luck. You'll do great out there." He rocked back and forth in his black dress shoes and I wondered if he was thinking about giving me a hug or a high five. Instead he performed a classic Aaron pivot, and chugged his arms getting his train ready to depart. Before leaving he flashed me his huge smile. Our eyes locked briefly, and in those seconds, all the electric waves surging through me collected as if pulled by a magnet and traveled on one current that connected Aaron's gaze to me. "Break a leg," he joked and walked back behind the curtain. A jolt knocked me backward as the electric connection broke. I stood trying to catch my breath and find my composure before my name was announced for my performance in the talent competition.

After my piano solo, I bowed graciously to the judges, smiled at the crowd, walked off stage and went directly into the dressing room to change into an evening gown and pin up my hair. The disposable armpit guards I had used to prevent sweat marks were completely soaked through. I tossed them into the garbage can and put new stain guards in my evening gown. Dodging clouds of hairspray, I twisted my hair and secured it off my neck with bobby pins. There were still five girls left to perform and I couldn't stay in that stuffy dressing room. My red sequin dress was cutting off my circulation, and I was choking on hairspray and glitter. I pushed open a backstage exit door and stepped into the cool air of a beautiful October evening. I should have thought before I let the door close and lock behind me.

I pulled the stage door, but it didn't budge. I retried, shaking vigorously. Locked. How could I be so stupid? Maybe the pageant was already going on without me. I knocked my knuckles against the steel and shook the handle with urgency, shouting for anyone to open the door. The only other way to get in was through the audience entrance, and I couldn't imagine walking up the aisle and passing the judge's table with a weak smile to get back on stage.

A window over the ledge was open a crack. Perhaps I could get someone's attention by calling through the window. I hoisted my dress and climbed up onto the ledge, pulling myself up to the window. "Hey, is anybody in there?" I called out. "I'm supposed to be in the pageant, but the stage door is locked." I heard the sound of the door open and released my grip from the window, balancing myself against the brick wall of the ledge and saw a head of slick brown hair poke out the door and look around.

It was Aaron.

"What are you up to?" I called down, trying to sound casual. "Aren't you supposed to be doing your escorting duties?"

Aaron looked right and left, finally realizing the sound of the voice was above him. "Yes, I am. And they've sent me to escort a certain escapee back to the pageant." He propped the door open with a chair and came over to where I was balancing on the ledge. "What are you doing? People are looking for you."

"Have they started the next round?"

"They are just lining up for evening gown," Aaron answered then looked puzzled at the situation. "How did you get up there?" he asked, looking up at me.

"It's called climbing, and it's not generally recommended when wearing shoes like these." I lifted my dress an inch to reveal a pair of spiky thrift store heels that I'd spray-painted and covered with red glitter. I stepped carefully along the edge, bracing myself to jump.

"Whoa. You're going to break at least one ankle if you do that," Aaron said.

"Maybe I could use a little help?" I asked, feeling embarrassed and wondering how to explain my predicament.

"Hold on to my hand." Aaron reached up and supported me while I got into a seated position on the ledge. "Now jump. I'll catch you."

I pushed off with my hands and jumped into his arms, never pausing to question whether or not he would catch me. The touch of his hands was warm against the cool skin of my back. He settled me onto the ground, but didn't release his hold around my waist. A tingle surged through me, but this time, I noticed that Aaron reacted, too. Usually suave and in control, his breath stopped and when he started to talk, he gasped a bit and his voice stuck in his throat.

"You look absolutely beautiful tonight," he said. He wasn't smiling. He was looking at my face as if he had never before noticed that my eyes are brown. Dark brown.

"Thank you," I answered, caught by the same wire of current from his eyes to mine. "You look pretty dapper yourself."

"Your music was amazing," he said. "I didn't know that you play piano." The weight of his hands on my hips was a sensation I'd never before experienced. His hold gave me weight that at once grounded me and gave me flight.

"Well, you'll have to give credit to my mother for making sure I practiced." In his hold I wanted to remain perfectly still, but stillness was a posture completely foreign to me.

Aaron blinked and shook off the connection. "I'd better get you inside. They'll be wondering where we are." Aaron opened the door, slid the chair out of the way and took my hand, guiding me inside.

"Thanks for rescuing me." I lifted up my dress and walked ahead of him through the door. "I didn't know how I was going to get back inside."

"Were you trying to run away?" Aaron asked.

"Maybe I was thinking about it."

"It's good you didn't." Aaron moved the chair out of my way. "All your adoring fans would be disappointed." He walked me to my place in the lineup before walking behind the curtain to wait across the stage with the other escorts.

When I stepped into the spotlight, I saw Aaron waiting at the center of the walkway for me. He must have traded places with another senator to be my escort. I walked out and offered him my hand, which he took confidently, then performed his classic pivot turn toward the audience and helped me down the faux marble staircase. Holding his hand felt brand new and anciently familiar. At the front of the stage, he gave my hand an encouraging squeeze before letting me go to turn circles so the judges could assess me from every angle.

At the end of the evening, after the points had been tallied, my name was announced as first attendant. I stepped forward, bending down to receive my banner and tiara. Aaron was on the front row standing, applauding, and whistling. He watched me with a look that said I was the most amazing girl he had ever met. Behind him Laiah was making notes, as I'd asked her to, on why I had come in second place.

AARON TOOK A different girl to every school activity and dance for the rest of the year, but he didn't ask me out. Laiah assured me it was for the best. "He's a massive flirt," she observed. The last week of school before Christmas break, I was cramming for finals when I saw Aaron walking around with a video recorder on his shoulder. He was making a movie, interviewing all the people he knew on campus, which was practically everybody. "Does that boy ever study?" Laiah asked.

The first day back from winter break, I was in the student council office eating a tuna sandwich when Aaron walked in like he'd just won a jousting tournament. "I am done with girls," he announced flinging his arms wide as if he had been liberated. "It's my New Year's resolution. I am not kissing any girls for the rest of the school year."

"What do you have against girls?" I asked.

"Nothing. I like girls, but they're distracting. This semester I am going to focus on my classes."

"I bet you won't make it one week," I challenged.

"I'll make it longer than you."

"No way."

"Every day you eat a sack lunch." Aaron pointed to my sandwich. "Tell you what. If I kiss someone before you do, I'll buy you a steak dinner."

"Deal." I felt pretty confident about winning. "We have to write it down and sign it." I grabbed a scrap of paper and wrote out the bet. "It's not valid until you sign it."

Aaron took the pencil out of my hand and scribbled his signature, ending with a dramatic underline. "Now, we shake on it." He shook my hand so vigorously that my tuna sandwich broke apart and fell to the floor. After dusting it off, I took a bite. Aaron raised his eyebrows.

"What?" I said. "Never waste a perfectly good sandwich."

Later, I replayed the incident for Laiah while we checked mascara at the bathroom mirror. She said, "You should not encourage that boy. He is too Don Juan for you. And he doesn't take school seriously."

I didn't see Aaron again for several weeks, not until after spring break and after debate nationals in Orlando. He cornered me coming out of the office in mid-April. "Congratulations, national champion. You look really good with a tan."

"These toes have touched the Atlantic Ocean," I said, pointing to my feet, which were clad in snow boots. Zipping my snow coat, I pulled the hood over my head. Outside we were getting pounded with a spring blizzard.

"Dinner, this Friday? You still owe me." He grinned widely.

"No, sir. You lost the bet. You owe me," I poked his chest for emphasis.

"I will buy dinner. You owe me your presence."

"I COULDN'T GET out of it," I told Laiah that night. "Besides, he's taking me to a *restaurant*. It's free dinner." After a week in Orlando eating catered meals, I was discovering a new world existed outside of tuna fish sandwiches.

"Go to dinner. That's fine. But don't let him go all Fabio on you. And don't do anything to encourage him."

When Aaron picked me up, I was wearing a plain brown, shapeless cardigan sweater and my Coke bottle glasses.

"I didn't know you wore glasses," Aaron said after the waiter seated us.

"I usually wear contact lenses."

"So do I." Aaron took the pitcher of ice water and filled my glass.

"I know. You wear colored lenses." I took a sip.

"No, they're not tinted. They're just regular, clear disposable lenses."

"Oh." I gulped ungracefully as an ice cube went down my throat. "Your eyes are so green."

Aaron smiled and handed me a menu. "Order anything you want."

I scanned the menu. "They serve liver and onions here?" I squealed.

"You like that?"

"Absolutely. My grandma used to make it. It's one of my favorites."

Aaron plugged his nose jokingly while I ordered. There would be no risk of a doorstep kiss with the smell of liver and onions on my breath.

I was wrong.

"Aaron Warner. I thought you weren't going to kiss any girls."

"Maleah Day. You are not *any* girl."

He kissed me again.

—❧—

THE VISION OF my perfect future had always included finding my handsome *Mr. Right* and adding several coordinating children, like acquiring an eight-piece set of matched luggage. It didn't happen for several more years (Aaron and I went different directions for a while, living in opposite hemispheres, in fact) but when we were reunited, I again fell for him just as hard and just as fast. When news of our engagement spread, one of our former professors said, "Together, those two could conquer a small country."

I thought, *Why stop with one country?*

In Aaron, I had found an equally driven—though far more spontaneous and fun-loving—man whose untamed entrepreneurial spirit had me convinced that we would, in no time, be the youngest couple to grace the cover of *Fortune magazine*.

CHAPTER 4

Overnight Failure

Thursday 1:20 p.m.

WHILE I DRIVE, I listen to Laiah's chatter as if my very existence depends on the presence of her continuous background babbling. She has me caught up in imagery and memory, to take my mind off these contractions.

"I haven't conquered the world," I bemoan to her. "I'm nearly thirty-one and I have nothing to show for my life except for all the meals I've cooked and the spills I've cleaned."

"You have Aaron and the kids." Laiah reassures, though she and I have had endless discussions about whether having children makes a woman successful.

"You know how people become an overnight success?" Laiah is available to talk and I've got nothing but wide time and an open road. "I feel like I got married, had a baby, and became an overnight failure."

WHILE AARON AND I were engaged, I imagined marriage would be a simple merger of our two life vehicles into one fast lane. We would slow down just enough to sign our marriage license, then hasten forward to finish school, find jobs, start our family, and achieve our wildly successful future. But our first year of marriage seemed to be one setback after another, and most of them my fault.

The moment I graduated from college, I took my double bachelor's degrees and scoured the job ads with picky arrogance expecting employers to line up outside *my* door begging me to come—and to please bring my impressive resume—to work for their company. But weeks of job applications and interviews wore down the point of my ambition. In the real world, nobody cared about my political science degree or my grade point average. In the end, I took an entry-level tele-sales job working alongside high school dropouts as a glorified telemarketer.

While Aaron finished his degree and worked retail at night, we thought it would be a great time to have a baby and start our own internet company. This was 1997 and buzz about the World Wide Web was breaking decibel levels. Giddy with possibility, Aaron and I signed our names on the dot-com line. We had discovered the path to our dreams, an enterprise we could run together from home. We had a computer that I'd won in a pageant, but the rest of the business investment required two things I thought I'd never do: break into my savings account and use a credit card. Figuring we'd have the investment paid off before the first credit bill came due, we purchased a combination color ink-jet printer/scanner/fax machine—cutting-edge technology—signed a rental contract on a pricey credit card service, and paid for a lease on cyber retail space inside a virtual mall called Galaxy Plaza. We met with our business mentor and began designing our very first website.

In May Aaron presented me with a wrapped box.

"I've never gotten a present on Mother's Day before." I read his homemade card: *To the most beautiful soon-to-be mommy.* I unwrapped the paper and lifted the lid. Aaron was so excited for my stomach to grow that he had bought me maternity clothes. "You are too cute," I said, giving him a kiss. "I'm the luckiest girl in the world."

By the summer, my tele-sales company had gone under. I was six months pregnant and unemployed. Our internet store had not made a single sale. And even though I was only twenty-six weeks along, I began to have contractions.

"We don't know what causes some women to actively contract early in their pregnancies," my doctor explained. "We also have no way to tell which contractions will lead to a premature birth and which are harmless." To be on the safe side, he prescribed Brethine, a drug usually prescribed to asthma patients, which was also believed to help slow down pre-term labor.

I asked my mother if she'd had preterm labor. "Oh, it seems I had a lot of pains with some of you kids," she said, but the doctors never put her on medication. She delivered all eight of us before epidurals and ultrasounds. And for some of us, before they allowed the fathers to be in delivery rooms.

I had expected mothering to come naturally to me, to know instinctively what I needed to do, but I ended up dragging Aaron multiple times to the labor and delivery unit, thinking it was real labor, only to be sent back home. Each time, as we left the hospital after the "false alarm," I felt humiliated. A woman should know when she's in real labor.

Danny was born three weeks early. A goop-covered, squished ball of flesh, he made his entrance holding tightly to his umbilical cord like a little bungy jumper hanging on for dear life. I looked to Aaron to see how I'd performed. His face was a mix of fascination, excitement, and a tinge of horror.

A nurse took Danny for his first real bath. She brought him back an hour later washed and bundled, but without the hospital cap on his head. The babies in my dreams had always been bald, so I couldn't have been more surprised to see my son with a head full of fine, dark hair styled into a handsome side comb, looking like a perfect gentleman in miniature. I accepted the warm bundle and brought him to rest on my heart. "Danny, I'm your mom," I said, trying the title on for size. "It's so nice to finally meet you." I unwrapped him like a Christmas present and examined every micro part of him, from his tiny toes to his itty-bitty ears. My mother had always said I would recognize my own baby, that my love would be instant. He felt strange and familiar to me, like a pen pal with whom I'd developed a distant relationship, but was just now meeting face to face.

When Aaron went home to shower and change clothes, I rested my head against the pillow of my inclined bed and watched Danny's belly rise and fall with each newborn breath. Now that the commotion had died down, I thought back about the delivery and wondered how I did. The nurse had left a folder of information on the stand. Sifting through the pages, I found information on breastfeeding, circumcision, immunization, and a chart to record each diaper change and the color of its contents. But where was my childbirth report card? What grade did I earn on my delivery? Had I been brave? Did I push effectively? How did Dr. Wimmer score me compared to his other first-time mothers?

I didn't hear a sound or a knock on the door, but when I opened my eyes Laiah was there. She moved around the room touching the equipment, brushing her hands across the machines before perching next to the hospital bassinet to examine the bundled package inside. "He's beautiful. How did the delivery go?"

The words spilled out of me. I wished I could do it over again. I regretted getting the epidural. I could have delivered without it. Childbirth was the biggest performance of my life, and I didn't even get a dress rehearsal.

"I'm sure you were fine," Laiah said. "I bet all women feel that way." She lifted the information card on the bassinet. "Danny Aaron Warner. Six pounds, seven ounces. Eighteen inches. Born at 4:45 this morning. Apgar score 7.5." She stretched her neck and tilted her head. "Why did he score low on his Apgar?"

"Seven isn't that low, is it?" I fretted. "They marked him down for being born a little early, for not crying loudly, for not moving a lot, and his coloring wasn't what they wanted. I've been sitting here thinking what I did wrong. What did I do yesterday that made my water break three weeks early? Did I miss a day taking my prenatal vitamins? Should I have let the landlord spray for spiders?

"You'll figure it out," Laiah assured. "They say mother's intuition is better than a medical degree."

"They did upgrade him to a nine on the Apgar after thirty minutes," I consoled myself. "That's not bad."

"No, that's not too bad. You'll score better next time."

I didn't have to wait long to get my "next time." When Danny turned four months old, I was pregnant again. Since my telemarketing job had folded, I had worked a series of dead-end temp jobs and we still hadn't seen an internet sale. With a wife and almost two children, Aaron figured it was time to stop playing wide-eyed, naive dreamers and plant our feet in the real world. He sent out his resume and was hired by Cloverman Financial to open an investment office in a booming Sun City retirement community northwest of Phoenix. We would be moving to Arizona.

Thursday 1:30 p.m.

My memories are interrupted by the all-too-familiar tug of uterine muscles. I hold my breath—which is not what you're supposed to do during contractions—until the pressure subsides. Expelling the breath, I collapse over the steering wheel, letting my arms hang heavy while the air conditioner blows the moist spots of my blouse. All around me the Sonoran Desert is rolled out like a brown picnic blanket disappearing into the sky as far as my eyes can see. Driving this desolate road reminds me of the day, nearly six years ago, when Aaron and I left Utah for Arizona. The angle of the sunlight on the aluminum sides of our U-Haul created the illusion that we were pulling a billowing covered wagon. Some of my ancestors had traveled the same stretch of road by wagon or on horseback as they settled the southern areas of Utah. I was not so different from those pioneer women, traveling with one baby in the backseat and another in the womb, following my husband to break ground in untilled soil.

In Arizona, we were too young to live in the age-restricted Sun City developments, so we set up our nest in the city called Surprise. The first story we heard claimed the town got its name when US President Franklin D. Roosevelt looked out from the window of his personal train, the *Ferdinand Magellan*—equivalent to today's *Air Force One*—and said something to the effect of "being surprised anyone lives here." Other folklore credits Flora May Statler, whose name appears on the town's first official subdivision documents. The tale claims that when Flora May signed the documents dividing one square mile into affordable housing for agriculture workers, she declared, "I'll be surprised if it ever became a town." The truth is far less colorful. It was Statler's husband, Homer C. Ludden, who named the land after his hometown of Surprise, Nebraska, in the same way that Peoria, Arizona was named by settlers from Peoria, Illinois. I know this because Peoria is where my sister, Annice lives—the Arizona, not the Illinois. One reason this move was exciting for me was that I would live close to my sister.

Annice and her husband Calvin were waiting in front of our apartment when our U-Haul pulled in. They helped us unload our hodgepodge of secondhand furniture including a folding card table we used as our kitchen table. When Aaron and Cal hefted the rickety hide-a-bed couch we affectionately called *the "floral beast"* Aaron said, "Let's take this straight to the dump." I told him to stop joking and put the couch inside because I didn't plan to buy new furniture until he was making consistent commission.

Moving in took all of two hours, but we were drenched hair to heels with sweat from working in the July heat. We unpacked our swimsuits and spent the rest of the night cooling off in the community pool and slept with all the blankets kicked off and a borrowed oscillating fan blowing full speed in our upstairs bedroom.

CHAPTER 5

Stay-At-Home Mom

ON MONDAY AARON left for his first official day of work. I walked him to his car and kissed him goodbye. "You'll be great." I smoothed the collar of his dress shirt and straightened his tie. "You look very professional." He drove away using wads of tissue to keep his hands from burning on the steering wheel. Aaron's car disappeared around the corner and I stared for a while feeling like a foreigner in a new land.

Inside the apartment I plopped down at the card table, propping the side of my head up with my hand. Danny tried to stuff Cheerios into his mouth at the same time I delivered a spoonful of rice cereal, and the result was a mosaic of oat circles pasted to his upper lip. I sighed. "It's just you and me, kid." I scraped a dribble of mush off his chin with the spoon and re-fed it to him. "What do we do now?"

My day was wi-*ide* open.

For the first time in my life I didn't have scheduled obligations— no job, no essays to write, no rehearsals, no upcoming competitions. Nothing in the world made me more uncomfortable than blank space on my calendar. Today, I was staring at a whole lot of blank space.

Aaron returned at 5:00 p.m. with a sunburn. His hair was matted and sticky. His dress shirt marked with sweat stains. For the next several months he would be knocking door to door introducing himself and trying to win new clients. "How was your day?" he asked, dropping his bag on the floor.

Should I tell him the truth? That I pushed Danny in the playground swing until we were both so hot and sweaty that we spent two hours cooling off in the pool, then when I laid him down for a nap, I also fell asleep for two hours? In one day at college I would have taken two tests, attended three meetings, written a paper, practiced two hours of piano, and talked to at least twenty different people. The whole day had passed and I hadn't *done* anything. "We had a good day" was all I offered. "How about you?"

I didn't exactly have a plan formulated when we moved to Arizona. My post-college attempts at launching a career had been a big strike out. It made the most sense to follow Aaron to Arizona, where he would start his career and I would figure something out along the way. We didn't want to send Danny to daycare, and besides, at six months pregnant, I wasn't an employer's most desirable new hire.

"I feel like a freeloader living off of Aaron's hard work," I told Laiah during our next conversation. He was burning his feet walking up and down every street in Sun City Grand, while I sat in an air-conditioned apartment with a nine-month-old who slept through the night and napped twice a day. Laiah and I detested the image of the bonbon-eating, soap-opera-watching housewife who lounges all day in a bathrobe and fuzzy slippers, while the husband labors to bring home the bacon. We had promised we would never become one of *those* women.

"Just make sure your marriage stays equal," Laiah advised. "An unequal marriage is unhealthy. Aaron needs to know you're working as hard at home as he is at work."

Laiah always had the answers to my dilemmas, but I was trapped in the apartment all morning and afternoon while Danny napped. I didn't want to be seen as just a stay-at-home mother, but what could I do in 1,100 square feet to work as hard as Aaron? How could I contribute to the family income without having to use daycare?

The answer was thrown at my door the next morning. The classified section of the *Surprise Independent* made my heart jump. There were hundreds of pianos for sale at amazingly affordable prices. In the heart of an aging community, the toll of arthritis, death, and downsizing were pushing pianos onto the street. With ten students, I could pay for a piano in two months.

"What if your mom teaches piano in the afternoon while you sleep?" I tapped Danny's nose. He gave me a tooth-and-gums smile. The piano arrived the next week with tuning included in the price of delivery. Flyers with my name and phone number were hung in the apartment office, the laundromat, the post office, and the grocery store.

My first lesson was exhilarating. Linda was a retired schoolteacher already proficient in piano who wanted to keep her skill polished. She paid me even though I said the first lesson was free. I pocketed the money with a sense of satisfaction at having accomplished something with my day. No bonbon-eating mooch would I be.

Life was progressing successfully until the first prenatal appointment with my new obstetrician. "You're twenty-nine weeks and already dilated," Dr. Magnuson said with a grim expression, asking a nurse to take me to labor and delivery for contraction monitoring. Two hours later he sent me home with a prescription and suggested limited activity and bed rest. After the appointment, I picked Danny up from Annice's house, told her the glum news, and drove reluctantly to the pharmacy. At the apartment I stared a long time at that brown bottle before twisting it open. The pills were tiny, but they were hard to swallow, mostly because neither Dr. Wimmer nor Dr. Magnuson were certain I needed the medication.

Both my Utah and Arizona doctors had told me that some women have preterm labor and don't deliver early while other women with preterm labor deliver premature infants. "The only thing we know for certain," they had both confirmed, "is that every week too early means several weeks in the Neonatal Infant Care Unit."

With my baby's health at stake, I set alarms to take the pills every four hours, even during the night. The medication turned me into a wild-eyed insomniac who shook around the clock like an addict going through withdrawal.

The next day I didn't take Danny for our morning stroller walk or push him in the playground swing. Floors did not get vacuumed and bathrooms were left un-scrubbed. We didn't go to the library, the grocery store, or the pool. I lay on the couch listening to four hours tick away on the clock while Danny crawled on the floor around me. This new routine of non-doing was okay for a solid three days before we both went stir crazy.

Aaron had been updated about my OB appointment by phone, but I don't know how much the news or the ramifications had registered. He'd accepted a volunteer assignment in our church as president of the men's quorum, which meant he spent every evening after work at meetings or helping people move furniture. He'd slam into the apartment after work, dash up the stairs to change into either a white dress shirt and tie, or jeans and work gloves. Rushing back out the door, he'd blow a kiss to my bed resting station on the floral beast. On my back I lay immobile, staring at the ceiling and wrestling with the conundrum of whether it would be okay to get up and wash the dishes. If I could wash the dishes, why not wipe the counters? If I could wipe the counters, why not mop the floor? If I could mop the floor, then...

One night Aaron came home about 10:30 p.m. and crawled into bed next to me. I'd hardly seen him for days. He lifted the covers and scooted in, wrapping his arms around me and pulling me close. For weeks our intimate contact had consisted of me squeezing antibiotic drops into his eye for a scratched cornea, an injury he acquired chopping wood for our church campout. In his hasty comings and goings, he had little knowledge of what I did or didn't do in a day.

I stopped his hands. "Dr. Magnuson said I have to limit physical activity."

Aaron pulled back. "What does that mean?" he asked, releasing his hold.

Was sex a forbidden physical activity? I didn't know. For a man, that might have been the first and only question he asked the doctor. I'd been so upset about having to take the medication and the images of having an underdeveloped baby that the question of sex wasn't a blip on my radar. But how could I say that to Aaron? Before I could formulate an answer, Aaron rolled over, wrestled his pillow until it conformed into the shape he wanted, and began to snore. I tossed back and forth uncertain which position I should choose. On one side, my husband. On the other side, my baby. Both sides lumpy with angst. Who to choose and who to refuse?

—⚬⚬⚬—

BEING STRUNG OUT on bed rest offered me ample opportunity to converse with Laiah. "*What are you doing?*" she'd ask. "*Lying on my back,*" I'd say. "*Lucky!*" she'd tease. She knew I was sick to death of people thinking bed rest was a glorious, doctor-ordered vacation. It was hard trying to decide what things to do and what things not to do. It would have been easier to go ahead and do everything that needed to be done. And it would have been easier to take Danny to the playground than trying to keep him entertained and out of trouble from the couch. Every day he stood at the front door and cried to go swimming. We read all his books until their spines gave out and I gained a new understanding of why they are called "bored" books. Danny grew ornery and Aaron hardly acknowledged me.

"I think Aaron's mad at me," I mentioned to Laiah.

"He *is* out burning his butt to make money while you sit in your *cushy* apartment picking at your cuticles."

"I didn't ask to be stuck in an apartment all day." If the floral beast was anything, it wasn't cushy. "What should I do? How can I prove to Aaron that he didn't get a lemon when he married me?"

Laiah had the simple answer. "Make sure Aaron knows that being on bed rest is *not* enjoyable."

Laiah's insight was brilliant. If Aaron's out knocking doors in scorching weather, then it's only fair that I suffer as much as he does. I couldn't allow myself to read novels or watch movies or our marriage wouldn't be equal.

She agreed. "You might be on bed rest, but you should still find some way to be productive."

What could I do from this couch to contribute to our family? I decided to become personally responsible for our debt—which, in addition to our defunct business investment also included Aaron's student loan, a car loan, my wedding diamond, and an emergency room bill. I gathered files and set up office around the couch. Aaron might be the bread winner, but I could be the bread saver. I would manage our budget so tightly, not a single penny would slip through unaccounted. I crunched numbers and made phone calls making sure we were spending as little as possible, so every extra dime could go to paying off debt. I filled a notebook with insurance quotes from every company listed in the phone book, comparing rates before Progressive ever thought of doing it for me. I transferred loans to credit cards with zero interest introductory offers and spent hours haggling with customer service representatives to waive transfer fees. I paid my dues by working myself into a frenzy about it.

When our first power bill arrived, I called customer service complaining there was a mistake because it said we owed *$383.19 for one month of electricity.* The agent asked about our thermostat and nearly choked to death laughing when I told him it was set to seventy-six degrees.

"Most people set their thermostats around eighty," he informed me. "In Arizona you don't cool for comfort, you cool for survival."

My budget only allotted $100 per month for electricity. The thermostat was immediately increased to eighty-one degrees, and I returned to the couch fretting over how to squeeze the other $283 from our account.

The apartment became a sauna. Danny woke from his naps drenched with sweat and sat in front of the door crying to go swimming. It was a toss-up which location was worse for bed resting. Upstairs my bed was soft, but the summer heat rose to the top of our apartment and stayed trapped in those small bedrooms with no ceiling fans. Downstairs was slightly cooler, but the wire springs of the couch dug into my back. There really was no comfortable position on the floral beast. This game would go on for five weeks, choosing the least unbearable place: upstairs on my bed in the boiler room or downstairs on the wiry couch. There was never a clear winner.

Each evening when Aaron returned home, I was indeed miserable.

CHAPTER 6

Alone

Thursday 1:45 p.m.

LITTLE BY LITTLE, the air conditioner has stopped blowing cold air. Aaron told me the car was overdue for a tune-up, another reason he didn't want me to drive alone. The sauna-like feeling takes me right back to that summer six years ago when I was pregnant with Kate and trapped on bed rest inside the apartment. Another tightening begins low in my abdomen and winds like a pair of boa constrictors snaking their way up around my torso in opposite directions and compressing with all their might. Laiah rambles on while my skeletal-white fingers try to hold the car steady.

"What is Aaron going to give you for your birthday next month?"

She thinks Aaron owes me an extra special gift this year because he never got me a different present after I made him return the digital camera he tried to give me last year. I'd told him it was too much money to spend on me. We didn't need a $400 fancy piece of technology when my Kodak film camera worked just fine.

Three minutes pass on the car's digital clock before the constrictors give their hardest squeeze and recoil, gradually releasing the pressure. Before I can recover, the pulling of another contraction rips into my abdominal muscles. I brace myself with gritted teeth and fight against the contraction, my spine arching into the seat in opposition.

What if this is it? What if the baby is coming now?

I glance around the car and notice there is only one plastic water bottle with about an inch of liquid left in the bottom—not nearly enough to deliver a baby. If these contractions turn into the urge to push, should I crawl into the back seat or get out of the car? If I prop myself up against the back tire, then the afterbirth would soak into the sand instead of ruining the car's upholstery. What about tying off the umbilical cord? I look at my feet. *Sandals.*

The peak of a new contraction pushes an odd hiccup out my throat which morphs into an awkward laugh as I think of the perfect birthday gift. Aaron can give me a vehicle emergency kit complete with a blanket, wet wipes, water, flares, *string, and pain killer.* That would be a practical gift I wouldn't have to return, but I need it today, not one month from now.

The contraction wrings stronger and a tsunami of agony crushes my organs. The pinching escalates and I make a shrill cry which echoes against the silence of the desert. But no one is around to hear me scream.

I WAS ALONE the week before Kate was born—well, alone with eleven-month-old Danny. Aaron had to travel to St. Louis for a week of training and final testing. He couldn't legally earn commission until he passed his licensing exams. Annice was out of town as well. She and Cal were in—of all places!—*Africa*, on a two-week safari. Before she left, she and I exchanged apologies.

"I'm so sorry I can't watch Ashley and Tyson while you're in Africa," I said.

"I'm sorry I won't be here to help you with Danny," she said right back. We were both shaking like autumn leaves, partly due to medication—me from my recently-doubled dose of Brethine and Annice from her malaria immunization—and also due to worry. She was going to be one hundred percent away from her children for two weeks; I was going to be one hundred percent alone with my children, hoping one wouldn't get sick and the other wouldn't be born. Our goodbye hug was tinged with desperation, my belly poking between us.

"Do not have this baby until I get back from Africa," Annice begged.

"Have fun in Africa and do not get eaten by lions," I answered.

The day Aaron left for the airport, he kissed me long and held me tight. "Who will you call if your water breaks?" he asked.

I hadn't made many friends in the two months we'd lived in Surprise. Bed resting in an apartment isn't exactly fertile ground on which to cultivate one's social life. There was Linda, my piano student, but she was an only child, had never married, had no children of her own, and I wondered if the baby thing weirded her out. But I didn't want to worry Aaron more than he already was. "Patsy from church said I could call her if I needed help."

His hand on my stomach followed the movement of our baby's kicks, like a little game of whack-a-mole. "Baby, you stay put." He shook his finger at my stomach. "You are gwounded to your womb," he said in his best Elmer Fudd impersonation. "Corporate office promised they would fly me right out if you go into labor. If your water breaks, get an epidural. That should slow things down enough for me to make it back in time."

I'm already in labor, I thought behind my brave smile. I closed the door after Aaron and a buckling contraction hit, dropping me to the ground where I arched my back and cried, "Can I get the epidural now, *please*?"

Laiah was also occupied that week, with what exactly I can't remember. Who could keep track of her projects and promotions? She was always going places, doing important things, meeting significant people. Though it was impossible for her to visit me in person, she always took time to talk. While Danny re-watched VHS cartoons, I lay on the couch and brainstormed with Laiah every conceivable scenario from delivering the baby while holding Danny on my lap at the hospital, to my water breaking at midnight and me delivering the baby in my apartment by myself. The last scenario was not ideal, but we both agreed it would save a lot of money.

Thursday 2:00 p.m.

THE GLARING SUN bares down through the windshield. Streams of sweat drip from my hairline into my eyes, mixing with tears and making it nearly impossible to see. My mind is battered with unknowns. If I have to pull over to give birth, how long before the air conditioner would run completely out of coolant? How long before the tank runs out of gas? How long will my cell phone battery last? If I'm out of signal, can paramedics find me? If this isn't I-10 to Tucson, how long before another vehicle will drive past?

When I was pregnant with Kate, imagining what I would do if I had to deliver alone in my apartment, at least I had water, towels, and air conditioning. If needed, I could have screamed loud enough for neighbors to come. Out here, who will hold the baby while I clean myself off? What if I need stitches? How long can a newborn survive in hundred-degree heat? Doctors are usually worried about a newborn dropping in body temperature, but what if an infant gets too hot? Breastmilk doesn't come in for several days. How long does it take a newborn to get dehydrated?

My mind grows bleary with images of a slimy newborn laid in the sand while I struggle to pack my torn perineum with wads of extra underwear from my suitcase. My overnight bag could work as a makeshift bassinet. Wiping the tears away from my eyes with my shirt sleeve, I fiddle with the car visor trying to block out the blinding rays, but it doesn't help.

A blurry scene appears in the distance. In the blinding glow I think I can make out a shape in the arid vista… It's a car, a Ford Taurus. The car appears to be abandoned on the side of the road; layers of desert dust have turned the once-gold paint to dull gray. Outside the car, a circle of buzzards perch, pecking at the dried-out carcass of a mother laying over her newly-born infant to protect him from the scavenging desert coyotes. The wind from my car speeding past blows the apparition into wisps of parched heat rising to the cloudless sky, but not before I see scorpions scatter out from the woman's ear and notice she is wearing my same floral maternity frock.

The long drive to Tucson gives the overtaxed faculties of a pregnant woman too much time to run wild. Next, in the barren distance, my weary eyes see the blue rectangle of a rippling swimming pool, one of those desert mirages with palm trees and a waiter carrying chilled drinks, served in a martini glass with a slice of lemon. How I wish I could take a break from driving and submerge myself in cool water, lazing on the miraculous buoyancy of weightlessness. Gazing longingly at the rippling image of my desert poolside oasis, I think how marvelous it would be to drive into that picture—the way Mary Poppins and the Banks children jumped into Bert's sidewalk drawing—and for the length of one musical number to *not* be pregnant, to *not* be contracting, to *not* be burning like Hansel and Gretel's witch in her own oven. For the duration of three verses and a chorus, I long to be a regular woman lounging on the side of a refreshing pool with someone else bringing *me* a drink. *Supercalifragilisticexpialidocious.*

⟞⟞ ⟋∿∿⟍ ⟝⟝

AS IT TURNED out, I didn't have to deliver Kate in my apartment on my own. Aaron arrived home on Sunday afternoon, and early Monday morning he drove me to the hospital. We stopped at Annice's house on the way to drop off Danny. She had been home from Africa since Friday. The night stars were still twinkling, and the orange sun was beginning to rise when Annice opened her door wearing light pajamas and fuzzy slippers. "Good luck today." She hugged me through the passenger window.

"I don't know if I can do this." My eyes were wet.

"There's no turning back now." She drummed the car door and turned away.

"Want to trade me places?" I called after her.

"Not on your life, sista! Hope you have a good epidural." Annice carried Danny's car seat—with him sleeping soundly inside—into her house and closed the door. I turned to Aaron and took a long, long breath. He laughed nervously.

After thirty minutes on the hospital monitors the staff prepped me for a C-section. The baby's heart rate was dropping with each contraction. They gave her a steroid shot to strengthen her lungs and they gave me Pitocin to speed up labor. I was fit to be tied about all the chemicals being pumped into me.

"I don't think I can do a C-section," I told Aaron. "I didn't come mentally prepared to be cut open." He squeezed my hand and told me everything would be okay, which might have made me feel better if he hadn't looked so worried.

"A C-section is the easiest delivery," our nurse tried to console me. She turned away and I could hear the words she meant only for herself. "It's the recovery that's rough."

I was able to deliver Kate without the C-section. When Dr. Magnuson pulled her out, he said, "She has the shortest cord." He held a meager length of umbilical cord and nodded for Aaron to make the cut. "The blood supply in the cord was getting pinched off the lower she dropped. That's why her heart rate was dropping."

I looked to Aaron to see how I'd done. He was cooing and kissing Kate. "Hello, little bitty. You gave us quite a scare." He looked as if we'd survived a near miss.

⸺⟅∿⟆⸺

REMEMBERING KATE'S TOO-SHORT cord, I realize something I hadn't considered yesterday during the argument with

Aaron. What if I can't deliver the baby on my own? What if I need a C-section?

Shuddering at the image of a shriveled, dried-out, dead baby, I pray with earnestness. *Please, God, send help. Please let another car drive by.* Suddenly my imagination shows a black van with dark windows pulling over behind my abandoned car. Considering the desolation of my location, I amend my prayer with a little more clarification. *And please don't let the vehicle belong to a serial killer hoarding an ax and duck tape, I mean duct tape. Please, let the next car belong to a retired nurse who happens to have a medical bag and morphine in her trunk.*

CHAPTER 7

The Longest Day

AARON'S TRIP TO St. Louis had been successful. He passed all his licensing tests and was able to move out of the backroom of a shared office and open his new office location in Sun City Grand. Kate was a few weeks old the day Aaron came downstairs showered, freshly shaven, and dressed in a new shirt and tie. "You look like a man with important places to go and people to see." I sat at our card table wearing wrinkled pajamas, my hair scooped up in a messy bun on top of my head, spooning oatmeal into Danny's mouth. Baby Kate was sleeping in the playpen next to the table and Danny kept pointing at her with questioning eyes. "It's Kate," I'd say. "Your sister." Danny would grin and drop a Cheerio for her.

Aaron kissed my cheek. "You're down here early." He sounded so chipper. I had fed Kate at 11:30 p.m., 2:30 a.m., and again at 5:00 a.m., and was craving a day of bed rest.

"Congratulations on your new office, babe. Your first day with a real desk and air conditioning. That's a big deal."

"Yes, it is. Have fun here. What are you guys going to do today?"

I didn't know how to answer. What did he think I *should* do today? What did he think I *could* do today? In between hooking a six-pound human to my chest every three hours and stopping eleven-month-old Danny from running over his new sister with his fire truck, what did he expect from me? Did he expect that all day I would recite the name of every dinosaur Danny brought me?

Because that's what I did. Did he expect that I would wince and cry each time Kate sucked on my cracked, bleeding nipples? Because that's what I did. Did he expect that I would lay Kate down on our bed and fall sound asleep next to her? Because that's what I did.

Each day I checked the mailbox for my report card from Kate's delivery, but it never came. Neither were there transcripts informing me I'd successfully passed Spaghetti 101 and could advance to Meatloaf 202. The mailbox did contain several certificates with Aaron's name written in gold calligraphy congratulating him on earning several licenses and showing his official titles. Those certificates got framed and hung on the wall of his new office. My bare walls could only mean that I wasn't succeeding at anything significant. Considering the fact that I hadn't even grown a sufficiently long umbilical cord and caused all sorts of panic and mayhem at the hospital, I figured my grade for Kate's birth couldn't be above a D-minus. I really needed to get my act together and start accomplishing something impressive.

———⟞ɤɤɤ⟝———

AARON HAD BEEN working from his new office for a few weeks when we woke one morning to find the windshield of our car shattered, a large rock resting culpably on the driver's seat. "Can you call the insurance company and see who they cover to fix that?" Aaron asked, exchanging for the other set of car keys. He drove away leaving me wishing I could trade places with him so I could spend the day in a clean office with my own personal assistant, and he could deal with the broken glass, two babies, and a claustrophobic apartment. I took a deep, deep breath before walking inside my apartment to face the day.

Strapping Danny into his booster seat, I gave him a pile of Cheerios and parked him facing the television before hauling the garbage outside to pick shards of glass from the car's upholstery. Kate was screaming from her crib upstairs when I lugged the vacuum back into the apartment. In the downstairs bathroom, I carefully took off my glass-speckled pajamas and scrubbed my hands, arms, and face before picking up Kate. Her tiny face was red. She looked indignant at being neglected. "I'm so sorry, baby girl." I laid her against my shoulder and massaged her tender back which was still covered in newborn hair soft as fur. "I'm here. I know you're starving."

Danny was kicking and struggling to get free from his straps. Balancing Kate, I struggled one-handed to release Danny's buckle and help him down. His soggy diaper was almost falling around his ankles, but Kate was crying to eat. When Kate finished, I resisted the urge to move her. I was learning that if I let her lie still for several minutes after she ate, without lifting, bending, burping, or jostling her, then she didn't spit up…as much. Once she was settled, I placed her and Danny on the carpet side by side, performing assembly line diaper changes. "What does Danny want to wear today?" I held up two shirts. He pointed to the one with green dinosaurs. No surprise there.

Locating the insurance phone number required a ransack of the office files, then I picked up the phone to find no dial tone. The internet was down, too. We'd have to go to the main office to call. In the family room, Danny was on his stomach nearly asleep in the middle of his pile of toys. "Hey pal." I shook Danny to wake him up. "No nap yet. Mom's going to take a quick shower, then do you want to go for a walk in your stroller?"

Danny perked up and pointed to the door. "Go," he said. I left the bathroom door open to listen for Danny while I showered. Out of the shower, I piled my wet hair into a twist on my head and attached Kate's car seat to the top of the stroller.

"Climb in." I patted to the bottom of the stroller. Danny crawled over and climbed into the storage basket. He didn't seem to mind that Kate was using his car seat or that he'd been demoted to the bottom stroller basket.

When I opened our front door, I was startled to see a woman with her hand up ready to knock. Sharon, our apartment complex manager, held a file with the name *Warner* on the tab. "I bet you were coming to pay your rent." Sharon smiled. "I thought it was strange you were two weeks late, but I can see you've been busy." Sharon gestured to baby Kate.

I'd completely forgotten to pay October's rent! "I'm so embarrassed," I told Sharon. "Let me grab my checkbook."

She stopped me. "Unfortunately, we can't take a personal check. At this point, it has to be a cashier's check. There's a $50 late fee, and we need it by 5:00 p.m. tonight."

After closing the door, out of habit I turned to grab the car keys, then remembered the broken windshield. I would be pushing the stroller to the bank inside the nearest grocery store.

"WELCOME TO SAFEWAY!" cheered a friendly, gray-haired greeter whose nametag read *Beverly*. The local grocery stores were staffed by no one younger than sixty. When Beverly spotted Kate in the stroller, I thought she might have a heart attack. Seeing a baby in Sun City was a rarity comparable to spotting a white rhino. She smiled so big she nearly popped out her dentures. "Everyone look! It's a baby!" In no time we were accosted as if we were the Beatles making a surprise appearance at Woodstock. "Let's take a peek at this baby." They circled the stroller. I opened the blanket so they could see all of Kate. "Oh, it's a tiny one. She's not very old." Danny poked his head out from beneath and looked up with a huge smile. The crowd stepped back as if a snake had wriggled out from a basket. "Oh, you've got another one hiding in there, too!" They looked unsure about a woman stuffing a live human into a stroller storage basket.

"He loves to ride in the bottom basket." I lifted Danny out and propped him onto my hip.

"Would he like a sticker?" Beverly's arthritic fingers made several attempts at unpeeling the sticker. She placed it on Danny's chest and rubbed it in three times. "There you go, son." Danny smiled. Beverly giggled. We finally made it inside Wells Fargo Bank with three helium balloons, free bakery cookies, a lollipop, and an *I Love Safeway* button. With the cashier's check in hand, I slid Danny into the stroller basket and hurried out of the store.

On the walk home, I kept tapping Danny with my foot and pointing out birds and airplanes to keep him awake. I needed him to nap at home. Kate grimaced and filled her diaper. I walked faster. The bare-windowed car was waiting for us exactly as we left it. I still needed to call the insurance company.

In the bathroom I stripped off Kate's messy undershirt, rinsed her in the sink, and started again with a fresh diaper and another outfit. I scrubbed the stain out of her clothes with a bar of soap. After Danny finished his hot dog and bread, I read him a short book and laid him in his crib. Kate was crying and hungry. I gathered a burp rag, blanket, and support pillow under my arm and settled into the recliner. When Aaron walked in for lunch, he found me sitting in the recliner with my feet propped up and *Charlie Rose* playing on the TV.

"Hi babe." He kissed my cheek. "Did you get someone to fix the windshield?"

Where had the four hours gone since he'd left this morning? "The phone wasn't working and I planned to go to the office..." I explained the late rent and the walk to the store.

"We can't leave it parked wide open like that." He picked up the kitchen phone and got a dial tone. Five minutes later he hung up. "A windshield repair company will be here this afternoon. Will you be here to pay them?"

I stared at him. He did in five minutes what I'd run myself ragged trying to do all morning. "I can't go anywhere with a broken windshield." I switched Kate to eat on the other side. "And Linda is coming for her lesson at 2:00."

Linda brought a floral bouquet, a note of congratulations, and a gift card to a baby store. I gave her a little hug. "These flowers are beautiful. That's so nice." During the lesson, Kate wouldn't sleep, but kept crying and spitting out her binky. I stood bouncing her on my hip while giving Linda instruction. "Play deeper into the legato and crescendo all the way until you lift your wrist at the end of the phrase." Linda stopped playing and looked with terrified eyes at Kate. I felt the familiar drip of milk running down my elbow and caught it with my hand before it hit the carpet.

"Oh my, your baby is"—she struggled for the right word—"leaking."

Had she ever seen a baby spit up before or did she think my daughter was broken? Kate made a familiar burping noise. I grabbed a blanket and barely caught the spray before it covered the back of Linda's shirt.

"Should I go?" Linda asked politely.

"No, no. It's okay. She does it all the time. She's a chronic spitter."

"Our lesson time is almost over anyway." Linda gathered her books.

"Next time we can play a few duets?" I called from the doorway as Linda used her cane to walk to her car. I hoped there would be a next time.

I closed the door and pulled the blanket away from Kate. Her outfit was drenched. Upstairs, Kate's clothes drawer was empty and the laundry basket was overflowing. "Kate, that was your last clean blanket and onesie. You can't keep this up. We are running out of things to wear." I changed my own shirt and snatched a onesie from Danny's drawer. It drowned Kate, but at least she wasn't naked. I made it downstairs in time for my next student.

It wasn't until I started making spaghetti for dinner that I realized I hadn't eaten breakfast or lunch. No wonder I was starving. I wanted to eat, but Kate was crying. I left the sauce simmering on the stove top and lifted Kate out of the playpen. "You're hungry too, aren't you little bitty?" The moment I'd popped out the footrest, settled in the recliner, got Kate positioned, and clicked the remote to the *Oprah Winfrey Show*, Aaron walked in. I was in exactly the same place I'd been when he came home for lunch. He eyed my relaxed position and leaned down to kiss my forehead. His skin was warm and I could tell he'd spent his afternoon knocking on doors again.

Aaron picked up the windshield repair receipt from the table. "Why so much?"

"I guess our car insurance doesn't include glass coverage."

"No, you have to request glass insurance separately. You didn't know that?"

I didn't recall any of my political science professors mentioning that certain auto insurance options were *a la carte*. In my fury to trim our monthly expenditures to bare bones, I'd moved our vehicle policy from one company to another, but didn't specify to keep the glass coverage. All the time I'd spent, the money I'd save in insurance premiums, was wasted with this repair.

The rent payment!

"Watch the kids!" I shouted to Aaron, pulling Kate off my breast. I reached into the stroller and felt for the cashier's check. I hooked my bra and adjusted my shirt while I ran across the apartment complex. The office was locked.

Walking back to the apartment, I saw Aaron driving out of the parking lot. I'd forgotten he had a meeting. He rolled down the window. "Danny is in his booster chair eating and Kate is in the playpen." He was on the street before I remembered to ask if he had quarters for laundry.

In the apartment, Danny had noodles hanging over his ears and red sauce spread on his face and down the front of his shirt. "Come here, messy boy." I lifted him out of his chair. "Let's get you washed up. We've got to make another trip to the store." Buckling the car seat bases back in the Oldsmobile, I found more glass buried in the seat and ended up vacuuming again. My stomach was cramping either from hunger or from doing so much twisting, bending, and walking. The simplest tasks seemed to take forever now that I did everything with two kids. I mostly needed quarters at the store, but as long as I was going, I might as well bring my coupons and get some grocery shopping done.

A man named Ed greeted us at the store entrance and decorated Danny with stickers. I pushed the cart up and down the aisles trying to think of what to cook for dinner outside of spaghetti and tacos. An elderly couple stopped next to my grocery cart. "Are these your children? My, you have your hands full…"

"Yes, I do. Full of good things." I coaxed Danny to make his duck sound for the couple. He performed on cue.

"Oh, that's so darling. Enjoy this time, they grow up fast."

"I will. Thank you. Have a good night." I tried to remember what I was shopping for.

"These kids need a balloon!" A Safeway employee with a curly clown wig stopped us and tied one balloon around Danny's wrist and one onto the handle of Kate's carrier. Our apartment would look like a birthday party.

On aisle seven, I was crouched down comparing the prices of mayonnaise when I heard a loud crash. "Danny! How did you reach that?" Stretching his little arms longer than I thought possible, Danny had pulled a jar of pickles off the shelf. I wheeled the cart to the front of the store and asked for a garbage and paper towels. First the windshield, now the pickles. How much broken glass could I clean up in one day?

The sun had set and the sky was dark when I pulled up to our apartment two hours later. "Okay, sleepy kiddos, let's get you ready for bed." My feet were exhausted and my arm muscles protested when I lifted Danny from his car seat. "Danny, you stink!" Kate also had poop up the back of the too-big onesie. I stripped her naked, washed her clean and opened her clothes drawer. Empty. "Oh no. The quarters!" In the midst of being the guest stars of the geriatric parade, I'd forgotten the quarters.

Once Danny was tucked into bed with a bottle, I carried Kate downstairs and collapsed into the recliner. It felt so good to be off my feet. My back ached, my head was throbbing. I couldn't remember if I'd had a drink of water all day. I helped Kate latch on and took out the remote. Just as the TV screen lit up, a key turned in the lock. Aaron was home.

"Hi, babe." I hastily powered off the television. "How was your meeting?"

"Long. I hate long meetings." Aaron noticed the heaping laundry basket sitting next to the door. "Did you want this washed?"

"Yes, but I didn't get any quarters."

He glanced at me and at the television. To him it looked as if I'd been sitting in this recliner all day while he was sweating in the hot sun.

"I did go shopping, but at checkout Kate was crying, Danny almost fell out of the shopping cart, I dropped the bag with the eggs, and I completely forgot to ask for change." The coupons, the sales, the balloons, the people…it had been too much for my brain. At one time in my life, I'd worked complicated calculus problems, and now I couldn't remember to get quarters from the store.

"I'll go grab some." Before I could respond, Aaron had his keys. He came home fifteen minutes later. I was still nursing Kate. He took the basket and headed for the laundromat.

"We're out of laundry soap," Aaron said when he came back with the empty basket.

"I know. I didn't have a coupon. I'm going to ask Annice to get me some when she goes to Costco."

Aaron looked through the cupboards. "Did you buy any Doritos?"

"No," I mumbled. "They weren't on sale."

Aaron headed up the stairs without saying goodnight, probably wondering why such simple tasks were so difficult for me. This had been the longest day. It felt like two weeks had passed since Aaron and I woke up and found the broken windshield. My body felt weary in a way I'd never felt before. My legs and muscles were achy.

Upstairs, everything was quiet. Aaron had fallen asleep. I craved a full eight hours of sleep, but I couldn't go to bed yet. I had wash going in the laundromat and I needed to give Kate her late-night feeding so she would sleep until 5:00 a.m. At least I could finally eat dinner.

In the kitchen I found that Aaron had put the spaghetti saucepan into the sink, squirted dish soap in the bottom, and filled it with water. In the bowl, the pasta had dried into hard noodles. Why hadn't Aaron asked if I'd eaten dinner before he ruined the sauce? Why wouldn't he save the leftovers? He knew how hard I worked to stretch our grocery budget. The more I thought, the more agitated I became. How could Aaron not notice that I hadn't eaten? There wasn't a dirty plate on the table next to Danny's, and there wasn't a dirty plate in the sink. Didn't he know that nursing makes me hungrier than an ox? I dumped the soapy water out of the saucepan, but it was no use, the sauce was ruined. The clang of the pan hitting the metal sink didn't wake Aaron like I'd hoped. The sound of his deep breathing, which I could hear all the way downstairs, cankered me with annoyance.

CHAPTER 8

Default

IN A FURY I slammed open cupboard doors putting away groceries, trying to wake Aaron, wanting to talk. I hated that to Aaron my life looked so easy—sitting in a recliner and watching television. I hated that he had no idea what my life was like. There was a time when I believed I was the most important person in Aaron's world. I believed he would anticipate my needs and come to my rescue, like he had in college, but I was ten feet below him and he had no idea that I was starving, exhausted, and hurting. That day I'd made sure everybody in my house had eaten three meals, but me? Who was in charge of feeding me?

I needed to talk to Laiah. She always seemed to be awake no matter the time of day and was always eager for a conversation.

"I don't impress Aaron these days," I complained.

"I'll listen," Laiah said. "Tell me something impressive you did today."

Late rent, botched insurance coverage, broken glass—today wasn't a good example.

"I'm still listening. Tell me something impressive you've done lately."

"I gave birth. In fact, I've birthed two babies for Aaron. Doesn't that count for something?"

"What push present did Aaron give you?"

"What's a push present?"

"It's the gift a man gives his wife for having a baby. Like Cal gives Annice a piece of jewelry, or your brother Vern gives his wife a Disney figurine. What did Aaron give you?"

Aaron hadn't given me anything. Push presents weren't in our budget.

"A lot of people don't view giving birth as an accomplishment. Women have babies all the time," Laiah pointed out. "There's no delicate way to put it. Getting pregnant and giving birth doesn't win you any trophies. It doesn't make you stand out in a crowd. It's not being a mother that makes you impressive, it's what you do on top of being a mother that makes you successful."

"So Aaron will never admire me as long as I'm just a mom?"

Laiah and I talked through most of Kate's late-night feeding until I had to switch Kate to the other breast. As long as she nursed on my right side, I was okay and could relax and close my eyes. But when I had to switch her to the left, my eyes started welling with tears in anticipation of the pain. She could never latch on as well on the left and the result was bleeding, scabbed nipples. I squeezed my breast and helped her take hold, wincing and crying as she sucked away. Writhing in the chair, trying to escape the shooting pain, to me those fifteen minutes were torture. When she finally released her suction, I sighed with relief and carried her sleepy weight up to bed, making no effort to be quiet. But Aaron didn't stir. He slept blissfully unaware of me, of the pit of hunger in my stomach, of the shooting pain in my breast, of the hours I was awake while he slept. His peaceful sleep taunted me.

I made it to the lower stair landing before crumpling to the floor and breaking into sobs, rubbing my eyes with the heels of my hand until they were raw. Still, Aaron slept. I couldn't stay in the prison of a house with him sleeping soundly, oblivious to my pain. Back upstairs, I searched through his pants pockets until I found the car keys.

The dark night air hung in thick curtains as I pulled onto Grand Avenue, the car pointed northwest toward Vegas. I didn't have a plan, but I figured there were plenty of jobs in Vegas and that casino owners wouldn't ask a lot of questions. With my one year of high school drill team experience, I could make it as a show girl, but I was not cut out to be a mother. Aaron would never find me in Vegas.

It took almost the distance to Wickenburg to realize I hadn't brought a wallet. Or shoes. Instead of driving five hours to Vegas, I turned around and drove in circles around Sun City Grand. A mangy coyote ran in front of my car. I panicked and slammed the brakes. It stopped and looked straight at me, its eyes glowing in the headlights. My throat was parched. I had no spit to swallow. My head pounded from dehydration.

I arrived in the Safeway parking lot for my third time that day. The automatic doors slid open to greet me even though I wasn't wearing shoes. Where was the greeting committee? There was no Beverly, no Ed, handing out stickers and cookies. Weren't there prizes for the mothers? The ones awake in the middle of the night?

The bottle of chilled Gatorade moved slowly down the conveyor belt. I could hardly wait to crack the seal and pour the thirst-quenching liquid down my throat. A droopy-eyed checker rolled it over the scanner. "A dollar twenty-nine," the man said sleepily.

I patted my pajamas, realizing—again—that I'd brought no purse or wallet. "Never mind." I left the Gatorade bottle dripping condensation and slouched out the door.

Driving home, I wondered what I would find when I pulled up to my apartment. I pictured all the lights on and Aaron frantically talking to police officers while Sharon and other neighbors stood gossiping in the glow of flashing red and blue lights.

When I turned the corner, the apartment was dark. Nobody had noticed I was gone.

I parked the car, checked on Kate, and walked to the laundromat to move the laundry from washer to dryer. At least I didn't have to deal with the embarrassment and shame of answering to police. Waiting for the clothes to dry, the actions of my evening began to sink in. *What mother in her right mind leaves her family in the middle of the night and heads for Las Vegas without shoes or a wallet? Was I going mad?* If Aaron knew, would he be afraid of me? I felt afraid of myself.

But on the other hand, how could Aaron not notice I was gone? I had made plenty of noise fumbling around our bedroom searching for car keys. Then I'd turned on a noisy engine beneath our open window, and driven away in our car and Aaron had slept through it all!

Perhaps enduring a police interrogation would have been easier than knowing the pain of that quiet truth.

THE NEXT MORNING, I was sleeping with Kate at my breast when I heard Aaron turn on the shower. Scenes of the night surfaced slowly, lapping like waves, my mind trying to decipher dreams from reality. Had Aaron noticed after all? Had he assumed I'd run an errand and would come back, so he didn't feel cause for alarm? What would I say when he got out of the shower and asked where I had been?

The sound of the front door closing woke me. I had fallen back asleep and Aaron had left for work without talking to me or leaving a goodbye kiss on my forehead. He didn't know, then, about my middle of the night drive, my almost trip to Vegas? He didn't know that a few hours earlier I had been meandering the aisles of Safeway in my bare feet. He must have assumed I'd lain next to him the whole night. Did he think my life was so easy compared to his because I was still sleeping this morning while he had to leave for a hard day at work? Did he have any idea while he stressed about gaining new clients and selling mutual funds that I was battling the unknown enemy of loneliness?

Kate had stopped nursing, leaving my bare breast exposed and a drizzle of milk pooling onto the sheets. I rolled into the wet milk, hit my pillow like a base drum, and added my own tears to the puddle.

—◦◦◦—

Thursday 2:10 p.m.

WITH ONE HAND over my eyes, I squint into the distance, scouring the horizon for any indication about where I am: a rest stop, a billboard, a road sign. I've never traveled to Tucson before, nothing about the surroundings is familiar, so how can I know if this is the road that will take me where I want to be?

Thinking back to driving past Phoenix, I recall seeing the baseball stadium. After that, was I supposed to exit or stay the course? The road, the contractions, Laiah's voice…it all blurs together. The contractions haven't let up. My body is exhausted. The fact that I can't remember how I got here is why I'm so confused. Was I paying attention? Did I consciously choose this road? Or did I get here by default?

—◦◦◦—

A MONTH OR so after Kate was born, one of Aaron's clients stopped by the apartment with a baby gift. She was a wealthy widow, dressed to the nines, wearing more jewelry on her neck and fingers than the sum total of what I owned. Aaron showed her into the apartment and offered her a seat on the couch. I was sitting in the recliner nursing Kate with Danny's head on my lap where he'd fallen asleep. Her eyes scanned the apartment—the kitchen, dining, and living space were essentially all the same room—paused on the card table and folding chairs we used as our dining set, then examined the floral beast. With great care, she sat gingerly on the very edge of a cushion and smoothed her skirt. "Where's the baby?" she asked at last.

"I'm feeding her. She's almost done." I pointed to the blanket draped across my body.

"Oh," the woman raised her brows and nodded knowingly, as if breastfeeding were a tribal ritual she'd read about in a *National*

Geographic magazine. "You must be Aaron's wife. And what do you do?"

The question caught me off-guard. *What do I do?* There was no nice, concise answer. How do I sum up my life? I'm a mom? No. That's not what she's asking. When people ask Aaron what he does, they don't expect him to say, "I'm a father." What do I do *outside* of being a mom? "I teach piano lessons. And I'm starting a song and dance group for kids called *Songbursts*."

"Oh, that's darling!" Her hair was perfectly coiffed; perhaps she'd come direct from the beauty salon. My hair was falling out of its pony tail. I'd broken down and gotten a permanent, my first since junior high. With two kids under age one, my hair had to be wash n' go.

"Where do you teach?" she asked.

I paused. Did she assume I taught in a music conservatory? "I teach here, in this room, while the kids nap."

"Oh," she replied as if the concept was very interesting. "So you stay home," she said triumphantly. At last she'd fit me in a category. Was that her impression of me? That I wasn't intelligent or capable enough to do something outside of home? That I stayed home because I lacked initiative to do more?

Aaron offered to walk her to her car. She slipped her arm through his elbow while I stayed here, firmly planted beneath two children, thinking about the past several months. The doctor said "bed rest" so I stayed home. Aaron went to St. Louis. Annice went to Africa. Laiah went...who knows where? I stayed home. All of my family came to see Kate; they left, and I stayed home. Tomorrow Aaron would leave for work and, again, I would stay home. Why? Because I have two babies who need to nap in their own beds and I don't want them to wake up to anyone else's face except my own. Is seeing my face enough of a reason to stay? With them? At home?

Laiah and I have always cringed at the term "stay-at-home mother." It's so overused, so cliché, yet this is exactly what I am. I had two babies and I don't want to use daycare, so I've become a stay-at-home mother by default.

A dictionary would describe the word *default* as a lapse of judgement, an overlook, or a mistake. But read the dictionary further and another meaning of *default* is a predetermined setting a device reverts to when no other alternative is selected. Clocks default to midnight. Calculators default to zero. Computers default to basic programming. Mothers default to caring for their offspring. We house, feed, and grow them within our bodies for nine months. Naturally we provide for their sleep, shelter, and food. This is a mother's instinct at its strongest. It's our default setting.

Did I choose to become a stay-at-home mother, or did I end up here by default? A default to tradition, religion, culture? A default to my natural instincts and inclinations? Was the decision to be a stay-at-home mother a deliberate and noble decision, a self-sacrificing decision, or a lack of decision?

How did I end up on this road? Did I take a wrong turn, or did I fail to take a turn? Was becoming a stay-at-home mother the best decision I ever made or the best decision I never made? Was I here at home by default or by fault?

Thursday 2:30 p.m.

I SCAN THE scenery again for clues to my location. When I told Laiah I needed to interrupt our conversation and call Aaron to ask directions, she let out an adamant *NO!* "If you call Aaron, he will ask how your contractions are, and either you'll have to lie or he'll talk you into turning around."

She's right, but what if I'm on the wrong road? For the past twenty minutes I've been praying with monk-like devotion for God to send me a sign. I'm not talking a heavenly sign like a choir of angels, nor am I asking for Moses to appear—though, of all the prophets, he has the most experience guiding lost people through the desert. I want a *sign*, specifically one of those green *road signs* reassuring I'm on Interstate 10 headed toward Tucson and not making a beeline for the Mexican border.

My heart lifts with hope as I spy a green form taking shape ahead. I breathe deeply, warily assessing if that twinge in my stomach muscles is the start of another contraction or just a reaction to the pressure of keeping my foot pressed hard into the gas pedal. I wish the cruise control was working. The green shape is speeding toward me and I slow a bit to read the words. My heart sinks when the green sign turns out to be a single barrel cactus, one branch bent to the road looking like a hitch hiker begging for a ride out of this desolate place. I'm so mad that I imagine driving straight into that cactus, exploding it to smithereens. Haven't I seen that cactus before? Though the clock says I've been traveling for nearly two hours, it feels like I'm covering the same ground over and over and over again, making zero progress. The scenery is so monotonous, every new mile looks exactly like the mile before. *Where am I? Should I turn around? Should I call Aaron for help or keep driving?* My life has become a continuous vigil, waiting for validation, for confirmation that I'm going in the right direction.

A new contraction pulls me inside out. I wish there were a way I could know if these contractions are the real thing or not. If I'm on the road to Tucson, I should be halfway there. This is my point of no return, my last chance to turn around. After this, if my water breaks and I call an ambulance, the paramedics wouldn't take me back to my hospital and my Dr. Woods, they would take me to the hospital in Tucson. I don't think I can endure pain like this for another two hours. I shouldn't be driving. I can feel myself caving in. The thought of calling 9-1-1 and riding toward a hospital and an epidural sounds wonderful.

Only one person can talk me off this ledge.

"Toughen up, girlfriend," Laiah tells me without apology. "Remember, this happens *every* pregnancy. These contractions *feel* real. They will rage for a few hours, but they *will* go away. You have to be stronger than your body."

"If this baby comes now, Aaron will never forgive me."

"You can go to the hospital and have this baby today," Laiah speaks with a do-what-you-want-it-doesn't-bother-me tone, "but I know you, and you'll regret it. You've talked for two years about getting your perfect childbirth. If you give up now, you'll spend the rest of your life wondering *what if?* and wishing for a do-over."

Laiah says exactly what I need to hear. She does the one thing that seals the deal and stops me from giving up. She re-tells me the story of what happened that Easter Sunday two years ago, when I delivered Tanner, my third baby.

CHAPTER 9

Tanner

DANNY WAS FOUR years old and Kate was three. We had moved out of the claustrophobic apartment and bought our first home, a corner house on the end of a street (and I'm not making this up) called Memory Lane. We lived on Memory Lane in Surprise, Arizona. Aaron's business had finally stabilized in the years following the tumultuous event of September 11. Life was good and we were ready to grow our family.

I was thirty-seven weeks pregnant when the phone rang during dinner and Aaron answered. "My parents are going to fly down on Friday. They both have a day off for the Easter weekend."

"The baby isn't due for three weeks," I reminded him.

He shook his head. "You're not going to make it three more weeks."

I gritted my teeth. *Yes, I am.* With help from a new doctor, I'd learned to somewhat tame the preterm labor. As long as I drank plenty of water and got off my feet when contractions flared, Dr. Woods didn't make me take the horrible Brethine medication. This pregnancy I was determined to carry full-term to forty weeks. "They are welcome to come, but I hate to have them miss meeting the baby. I'm not going to go to the hospital just because they're here."

Saturday morning Grant and Helen joined us at the Surprise Spring Training Stadium for the city's annual Easter egg hunt. The perimeter of the ball field was packed with parents and kids holding baskets and waiting for the Easter Bunny, who was standing on the pitcher's mound, to signal the start of the egg hunt. Aaron and I were lined up with Danny and Kate on the dirt beyond center field. There must have been twenty thousand people in the park. "This is ridiculous," I told Aaron. "I guarantee there will be at least twenty lost kids when this is done."

The bunny dropped its arms and the kids shot off like cannons. Kate sprinted for centerfield, outrunning the other three- and four-year-olds. In no time, the green field was dotted with hunched forms picking through the grass for prizes. Panting and holding on to my round belly, I ran behind Kate, trying not to step on eggs, candy, or children's hands. At last the buzzer rang, indicating the end of the hunt for this age group.

"Come with Grandpa. I'll take you to ride the train." Danny and Kate grabbed Grant's hands and followed him up the stadium steps.

Aaron's mom put her arm around my shoulder. "You doing okay?"

"I'm fine." I had sweat stains in the arms of my pink striped maternity blouse. The elastic waistband of my white capris was drenched. "Let's go stand in front of that giant fan."

AT 10:00 THAT night the house was quiet. Aaron's parents were asleep in Kate's double bed and Kate was in with Danny. I lay next to Aaron, trying not to move despite the war raging in my abdomen. After an hour, I slipped out of bed gripping my stomach and padded softly past my in-laws' room. I went to the farthest corner of the house and exhaled loudly.

"Ow. Ow. Oweee." I squatted, bent over, stood up, stretched my back, twisted, jogged in place—anything to ease the pain. The hands of the clock ticked slowly past midnight. I drank water from the kitchen sink and used the sprayer to cool my face. The pains didn't stop. A contraction pulled long and hard and something opened up down there. Kneeling on my knees, I banged my head against the floor, "Okay. I'll go!" Aaron's parents would get to meet this baby after all.

The hospital clock showed 2:25 a.m. when Delores greeted us at triage. Aaron sported jean shorts, a T-shirt, and four-hour bedhead. His eyes still wanted to be closed in sleep.

"Has your water broken?" Delores asked. I shook my head. She helped me onto a bed and strapped on the contraction monitors and checked dilation. "You are definitely in labor and are measuring five centimeters. We'll let you labor some more before calling the doctor. Do you want to stay in bed or walk around?"

"Walk around!" Aaron and I said together. Delores unhooked the monitors. Aaron guided my feet into slippers since it was hard for me to see my feet and helped me off the bed.

"So, what do you want to talk about?" I asked Aaron on our fifteenth lap around the nurses' station. Every other room was open and empty, I was the only patient here on Easter weekend. "Delores, who is the doctor on call tonight?"

She glanced at her schedule. "Dr. Babich."

I'd never heard of Dr. Babich. It had never occurred to me that one of the five doctors from my practice wouldn't be on call over a holiday weekend. I didn't want to be delivered by a complete stranger.

Tired of the hallway, Aaron and I retreated to our room and paced like caged cats. Not ready to be strapped to the bed again, I decided it was time to try the jetted tub. When Aaron and I toured this newly-constructed women's wing of the Del E. Webb Memorial hospital a few months earlier, our tour guide had boasted about the jetted tubs and DVD players with Bose sound systems in every room. We marveled. It was like a resort for bloated women.

Might as well get our money's worth.

"Why don't you lie on the bed and try to get some sleep," I suggested to Aaron, closing the door to the bathroom. The guide had not exaggerated—the tub was indeed deep enough to submerge a pregnant belly. My head dropped back against the porcelain edge and I drifted in and out of sleep as the warm water bubbled and massaged my raging muscles.

A KNOCK ON the bathroom door woke me up. "I'm Tina, your nurse for this shift. You've been off the monitors for several hours. I need to hook you up and check you."

I stood up and the water level lowered by half. Toweling off, I examined my protruding profile in the mirror. This is the largest my stomach would be. "Well, baby, are you ready for this?" I rubbed my stretched skin wondering if, in a few hours, Danny and Kate would have a *brother* or a *sister*.

While I was in the tub, Aaron had stayed in the hard chair. "You could have gotten on the bed," I told him.

He shook his head. "That would be weird."

I climbed onto the bed and let Tina strap me down. Twenty minutes passed and the monitor had not registered a spike or a flicker. Tina readjusted the straps. "Are you feeling contractions?" she asked.

"Not since getting into the tub."

Tina checked my dilation. "You're still a five. You've moved maybe one-eighth of an inch."

Before I sunk into that tub, I had been in full breathe-through-the-contractions labor. Now I had the relaxed, jiggly stomach of a sumo wrestler. That was good. I could wait one more day and come back tomorrow when one of my own doctors would be on call.

"Sorry to disrupt your peaceful night." I sat up searching for the Velcro on the straps. "It's hard for me to know when it's the real thing." I turned and hung my feet off the bed. "Aaron, honey, will you hand me my shoes, please? Tina, you have been marvelous. Thanks for everything. I guess we will go home."

Tina explained that hospitals have policies. "Because you're dilated to a five, I can't release you without a doctor's signature."

"I'm the only woman here on Easter Sunday. I'd hate for Dr. Babich to make a special trip for someone who isn't his own patient. I'm okay. I can come back tomorrow when my regular doctor is in."

Tina shook her head. I looked at Aaron. He shrugged.

"You don't have to stay on the monitors if they are uncomfortable," Tina offered. "Just let me know if you start contracting again." She left the room and closed the door.

I sat on the bed staring at the floor. My stomach was peaceful. I wanted to go home, go to church with my in-laws, celebrate Easter Sunday with my family. I didn't want to be stuck in this room like a hospital prisoner. Slowly, I turned my head to look at Aaron through the corner of my eye. I knew he was miserable. In six years of married life, Aaron had not once gone with me to see a movie in a theater because he can't stand to be stuck in one place for so long. Now, because of me, he was trapped in an eight-by-eight room. I swung my feet back onto the bed. "You can go home," I told Aaron. "There's nothing for you to do here but wait."

"I'm not going home." Aaron crossed his leg over his knee and steepled his fingers. "Let's wait for the doctor."

The silence ticked slowly.

"Do you want to watch a movie?" I offered.

Aaron walked out to the nurses' station and returned with a shrug. "They don't have any DVDs."

The tour guide had failed to mention that at 2:00 a.m., when I was hunched over in the passenger seat racing for the hospital, I should remember to stop by Blockbuster and select a movie or two.

Aaron pointed the remote at the wall-mounted TV and clicked through the selection of Sunday morning programming: televised evangelism or golf.

Finally I pretended to need ice chips from the hospital cafeteria so Aaron could walk around. While he was gone, I dialed Laiah. "Poor Aaron." She clicked her tongue.

"I wish I had been stronger," I cried to her. "I wish I would have toughed it out through the night. Aaron could be home in bed sleeping. Instead, he's stuck in a hospital waiting for a doctor to show up and there's not even a baby coming. It's humiliating that I can't tell the difference between real and false labor."

After talking with Laiah, I phoned my cousin who had recently retired from working at this hospital as a labor and delivery nurse. She had worked with all of the doctors. When I asked about Dr. Babich, I heard a catch in her throat. "Dr. Woods is my favorite. He's so good." Then, as if trying to reassure me she said, "I'm sure Dr. Babich will be fine."

Dr. Babich wandered in about 3:00 that afternoon and lackadaisically slid his hand into a glove. His tongue was blue like he'd been licking robin egg Easter candies. He didn't seem happy to be there.

My status had not changed. "I'm sorry you had to come to the hospital on a holiday," I said to Dr. Babich. "Anyway, thanks for signing the release forms. Now we can all go home and forget the whole thing ever happened."

Dr. Babich gave me a look that said *I did not drive all the way into town to turn back around. I am going to deliver a baby and make some money today.* Then practicing good medical school diplomacy, he said, "I can send you home, but you'll be back tonight and I will still be the doctor on call. Or I can break your water now and you'll have a baby by 5:00."

What I wanted was to go home and come back tomorrow when Dr. Woods would be on call, but Aaron said, "You might as well while my parents are here to help with the kids." He didn't want to repeat the scenario again tonight.

Dr. Babich chimed in, "You are in labor, you've just stalled. Breaking your water will get you started again." Since he was the one with the medical degree—and because I didn't want an angry, resentful doctor delivering my baby if I ended up back here at midnight—I agreed.

I'd never had my water broken before. The nurse handed Dr. Babich a tool which looked like a plastic crochet hook. Thank goodness he came all the way to the hospital to perform a procedure comparable to popping a balloon. If you hired someone to pop a balloon at a birthday party, you might pay them a nickel. Give the same effort a scientific name like *amniotomy* and you can charge megabucks and make people wait for hours like caged canaries for you to do it.

In the meantime, I got an epidural that nearly paralyzed me for life. Aaron fled to the furthest corner of the room and hid his face in his hands, peeking occasionally through his fingers to see if I was dead yet. The anesthesiologist inserted, pulled out, and reinserted the epidural needle four times. "You're so skinny, there's no fat to stick the needle into." I didn't find this to be an appropriate time to comment about my boniness.

Suddenly, with a five-inch needle searching its way around my spinal column, I felt my entire abdominal area expand, like someone had opened an umbrella inside my pelvic bones. At that moment everything on the inside of me urgently wanted to get outside of me. "Stop the epidural. The baby is coming!"

"Too late to stop now." The anesthesiologist was not going to let this bony specimen get the best of him. "I'm almost finished."

Tina dropped on top of me, bracing my shoulders in the gentlest tackle ever administered. "DO NOT MOVE! You have to hold completely still," she told me, then she shouted to the hallway, "Call the doctor." She couldn't make the call because she was holding me in a half nelson. "Keep still. He's almost done."

Eternity elapsed before the anesthesiologist withdrew the needle and taped the tubing against my back. Tina rolled me onto my back carefully. "Ow." I winced as the epidural entrance rubbed against the sheets, followed by more opening and something hard and round trying to squeeze through a hole ten times too small. "I can feel the baby's head!"

"Don't push. We have to wait for the doctor to get back." Tina supported my shoulders.

Seriously? He broke my water and left the hospital?

"Lay on your side." Tina helped me roll to my side. "Be strong and keep your legs together."

She should have told me that nine months ago.

"Does no one believe me? I. Really. Have. To. *Puuush.*"

Everyone in the room—except the anesthesiologist. He'd disappeared faster than a cub scout who'd broken the cookie jar—screamed in chorus: "DON'T PUSH." This included Aaron. Whose side was he on anyway?

When a woman has the burning need to push, telling her not to push is like exploding Hoover Dam and telling the water to stay put. "We don't need the doctor," I pleaded. "I trust you, Tina. You deliver this baby." I thrashed around on the sheets.

"No, no. They don't like us to do that." She patted my head. "You can hold on. He's on his way." Tina put her hand over my ear and screamed, "Did anyone get through to Dr. Babich?"

Was anybody even out in that hall? Finally, a desk clerk, or maybe a janitor, poked his head in the door. "He says he's checking out at Walmart and will be here in ten minutes."

Walmart? No one ever checks out of Walmart in ten minutes.

"Aaron, honey." I looked up, grimacing. I needed to push more than I've ever needed to do anything in my entire life. "One push and this baby will be here. You can catch it. I trust you."

Aaron backed into the corner waving his hands in front as he retreated. "No, no. Wait for the doctor."

Enough with waiting for the doctor.

Tina rubbed my back. "This will sound strange, but if you curl into a fetal position, it will help relieve the pressure." I tucked my legs up to my big belly pretending that the lower half of my body was not attached to the upper half. "Remember to breathe," Tina encouraged.

I inhaled. A soothing numbness spread from the center of my spine outward like a ripple. The epidural medication was kicking in, erasing the urge to push.

"The doctor is on the elevator." The janitor/clerk stood in the door holding a phone. Tina opened a cupboard and grabbed a surgical gown and gloves. The janitor/clerk helped Tina stretch out the gown like a ribbon across a finish line. "He's on the floor. Get ready, and in five...four...three...two..."

The door swung open and Dr. Babich walked into the gown and gloves, crouched down, looked side to side, and yelled, "Go."

That was my signal to snap the ball, but I couldn't believe what I'd just seen. Did Dr. Babich bypass the sink? What happened to official scrub-in policy? I didn't let my own husband touch me if he didn't wash his hands after shopping at Walmart. If I weren't such a lily-livered coward, intimidated by his medical degree, I would have asked him to turn back around and scrub. With soap. Instead, I stared.

"Go ahead. Push." Dr. Babich was giving the orders now.

I had just mastered *not* pushing and now he wanted me to push! Feeling strangely floaty and heavy at the same time, like a concrete cloud, I gave a wimpy push.

"No. Wait for a contraction. Push during the contractions." Dr. Babich rolled his eyes like I was the biggest idiot excuse of a delivering mother he had ever seen.

"I can't feel when I'm having contractions." My abdomen was as still and peaceful as a glass lake with no wind. The epidural was working, and I had found my happy place.

"I'll tell you when you're having a contraction." Dr. Babich watched the monitor. "Now. PUSH!"

"I am pushing."

"Push harder. Come on. Put some determination into it."

My determination skipped town about the time I realized we hadn't brought any DVDs. Ten minutes earlier I could have sneezed the baby out. Instead, we endured fifty-five minutes of everyone yelling at me to push harder and me shouting back, "I am pushing...I think...I can't really tell. Will I ever be able to feel my legs again?"

"It's a boy!" Dr. Babich declared, making note that the time of delivery was exactly what he'd predicted. He stood up from stitching, and I imagined I looked like a kindergarten class' first patchwork quilt project. At this point, when one would expect a hearty "Congratulations!" Dr. Babich gave me a look that seemed to say *The nurse will give you the information for direct deposit to my bank account. Holidays are double time.* Then he looked in the mirror, wiped blue powder off his mouth, and disappeared into the hall.

The epidural had been stronger than Schwarzenegger on steroids. My legs were cinderblocks. Aaron helped to balance the baby on my chest. He was tiny, six pounds seven ounces. "Hello there, Tanner." I traced the shape of his nose and cheeks while he blinked his eyes. My heart sprung wings which reached out and engulfed him. "Welcome to this big, wide world. I'm so happy you made it here."

I couldn't believe how much I loved him already. The ordeal was over. He was beautiful and perfect, so why was I wishing I could do it over again and do better? Why did I cave in and come to the hospital? If I had held out through the night, I wouldn't have missed Easter Sunday with my family. Aaron wouldn't have spent his holiday stiff and bored in a hospital chair. Dr. Woods could have delivered; he had a reputation for letting women stretch naturally and he tried not to cut episiotomies. Because I couldn't hold on a little longer, I was leaving the hospital stitched from belly button to back. The stitches rubbed and irritated. The very movements required to care for a newborn are the exact motions which exacerbate the incision site of an episiotomy. *What is that cruel irony, Mother Nature?*

CHAPTER 10

No

Thursday 2:45 p.m.

A DOOZY OF a contraction socks me in the gut and threatens to snap my spine in half. I desperately want to pull over and turn around.

"Hold on." Laiah does not waver. "Wait it out a few more minutes. This is exactly what you do. You have a series of back-breaking contractions for several hours, then they go away for a day or two, then they come back, then they go away. You are in this game for the long haul. There is no relief pitcher here. It's going to be on and off like this all the way to forty weeks. You can make it."

Remembering Tanner's birth—the jetted tub, the stalled contractions, the worst episiotomy—I press the gas pedal to the floor hoping to close the distance between me and the Tucson hospital as fast as possible. These contractions can't be any harder than the ones that took me to the hospital with him, and those went away. I have to be brave and stop second-guessing myself. I've been through this before. "These contractions are not real," I chant and bounce up and down in the driver's seat. "The baby is not coming now. These contractions will go away."

Here's a confession: When I registered for this conference I knew full well I would be thirty-seven weeks pregnant—I own a calendar and can do basic math. After Tanner's delivery, I wrote out a plan for my perfect childbirth scenario: 1) Go to the hospital at the right time, meaning the contractions are real and won't stop. 2) No doctor cheats, no medical intervention such as Pitocin or water breaking. 3) No epidural. 4) No episiotomy. 5) Make it full-term to forty weeks and deliver at least a seven-pound baby. Achieving this perfect birth plan and enduring the brutal contractions my body likes to throw at me the last weeks of pregnancy would require a big distraction. This conference was the perfect excuse to get me far away from a fretful husband, telephoning mothers, and the remotest option of a simple drive to labor and delivery for an injection of Pitocin followed by a lovely epidural. Making it forty weeks will require more willpower than I've ever mustered, but with this baby I am going to do *everything* right. I don't want any regrets, only the euphoria.

Please make these contractions go away, I pray. I just need to make it to my hotel in Tucson so I can recreate the jetted tub experience from Tanner's birth by taking a hot bath in my room. That should ease these labor pains. Swallowing a huge breath and a renewal of determination, I hit the gas and speed forward, hoping this is the right road to Tucson.

—◈—

AFTER BRINGING TANNER home from the hospital, Aaron and I struggled to find our groove. With two parents and three kids, we were outnumbered. We felt completely off-kilter until a miraculous thing happened. In July, Annice and Calvin went to Hawaii and left their three kids at our house, making us parents to six kids under the age of nine. Annice showed up one week later with a gorgeous tan. I hadn't brushed my teeth in seven days. Going from six kids back to three rebooted our system, and from then on, Aaron and I found a good rhythm balancing our own Danny, Kate, and Tanner.

Life became so good that in the fall, Aaron went back to night school to earn his financial planner certification. Danny and Kate both started preschool and Tanner was such an easygoing little guy, that those two free hours every Monday, Wednesday, and Friday felt like worlds of time that I couldn't leave empty. Aaron introduced me to one of his clients, Bob, who was looking for a part-time advertising sales rep and writer for his magazine. A perfect outlet, I thought, a way to keep my intellect sharp and get out of the house a few hours a week. Bob's wife, LuDene, volunteered to babysit Tanner for free and shower her grandmotherly love all over him.

The whole scenario was ideal, but I ran the idea past Laiah just to be sure. "Do you think I'll be able to handle three kids, piano lessons, and a part-time job?"

"If Aaron brought it up, he must think you can do it," she replied.

In a short time, it was obvious the job situation wasn't ideal. By the time I buckled three kids into my car, dropped them off to different locations, and drove twenty minutes to my sales area, I had forty minutes to contact business clients before it was time to pick up Danny and Kate from preschool. "You're always the last mom here," they would complain, the sweat dripping down their faces from waiting outside for me.

After two months, I told Aaron I needed to quit. "It's too much. I'm always late for preschool pick up. Tanner doesn't get a good morning nap. The kids are cranky. When I started working for the magazine, Tanner stopped sleeping through the night. I don't think he's getting enough milk. I'm tired. I'm falling asleep during piano lessons."

"You're the one who wanted something to do," Aaron offered.

When I told Bob my decision he said, "I wondered how you kept it going so long."

After that I decided to slow down. Three kids took a lot of time. I needed to make a conscious effort not to overschedule myself. And I needed to learn to use the word no.

In December, Aaron asked if we could have his client Christmas party at our house.

"No," I said.

"Why?" he asked.

"Because our house has only secondhand furniture and I have no idea what to cook for retired millionaires who have dined in the best restaurants around the world."

"It wouldn't have to be fancy," Aaron argued.

I held my ground.

A week after I declined hosting the client party, Aaron said, "Let's drive to Utah for Christmas this year."

"No," I said again.

"Why?" he asked.

"Because it's been four years since we stayed home for Christmas. I want to have our own family Christmas at our own house where we can open presents and play with toys all day and never change out of our pajamas. I want to relax and enjoy Tanner's first Christmas."

"You can relax in Utah," Aaron answered.

I stood my ground.

It was one of my favorite Christmases, watching Tanner roll around in the wrapping paper, laughing at its crinkling sound. For me the day was relaxing, but Aaron was fidgety, needing somewhere to go, something to do.

My schedule after quitting the magazine became more manageable. Sure, life with three kids was busy, but it was doable. That spring was one of my favorite times. The kids and I played on the playground at the park, fed breadcrumbs to the fish and ducks, went to library story hour, read hundreds of books, and swam at the city pool. I kept the kids busy and entertained in the morning so they would relax and watch movies while I taught piano lessons in the afternoon. Before my students arrived, I made sure to start dinner and tidy the house so that when Aaron came home from work the house was clean, the kids were contentedly playing, and dinner was in the oven. Life was good, but there was a problem: My life looked too easy.

―――⁂―――

THE NEXT SUMMER, Aaron and I attended a formal awards banquet hosted by Cloverman Financial.

"You ready to go?" Aaron called into the bathroom.

I came out wearing a black cocktail dress after spending an hour styling my hair and applying extra makeup. "Do you think this is fancy enough for tonight?" I fretted.

Aaron nodded. "You look beautiful. I'm a lucky man."

"I haven't worn heels this tall in a while." I tipped my foot, displaying my shoes. "I'm out of practice."

"Well, we'll have to get you back into practice by dancing." Aaron took me in his arms and swung me around the bedroom. He twirled me, dipped me, and planted a warm kiss on my mouth.

"Congratulations, Top Producer." I looked into his eyes. "You've worked hard this year. You deserve it."

The mood dropped and he lifted me to my feet and let go. "I hate that it's always about money."

At the banquet hall, we found our name cards on the furthest back table. We would have a long walk to the stage. I hoped my heels would hold up. We chatted with the other couples at our table over prime rib and shrimp. I'd been to enough of these to know the routine. Aaron's company is big on families. When Aaron interviewed for the job, they interviewed me as well. Traditionally, when a broker receives any recognition, the broker *and* spouse walk to the stage and accept the award together in a gesture that says, *I couldn't have done this without my spouse. This award belongs to my better half more than it belongs to me.*

When the waiter brought out dessert, the regional director stood at the microphone to present the awards.

"Is your chair broken?" the man on Aaron's right asked, noticing him shifting back and forth.

"No, I'm just fidgety," Aaron answered, embarrassed. Awards were given in order of sales production. When Aaron's name was announced, every person in the room would be able to guess almost exactly how much money he made. He hated it.

The emcee called names and brokers escorted spouses by the hand to the stage where together they accepted a plaque and posed for cameras.

"For our final awards," the emcee announced, "we are happy to introduce our five top producers."

That was my cue. I took a drink and swished the water to clean my teeth, applied a fresh coat of lipstick, fluffed the back of my hair, and smoothed my bangs.

"Aaron Warner," the emcee called into the microphone.

Scooting my chair from the table, I took a moment to smooth my skirt and prepare myself to walk in front of all these people without stumbling in my three-inch heels. I stood up to see Aaron practically jogging to the front, his eyes focused on the floor, already halfway to the stage. A low sound of whispers and giggles rumbled through the room. Aaron stopped and looked up. The emcee pointed to me. Aaron turned around, following the audience's hinting head gestures until he saw me, slowly retaking my seat. He whacked his forehead. I waved for him to go on without me. The last thing I wanted now was to be put on display as the most forgettable woman of the night. For a few seconds, Aaron went back and forth: go to the stage or come for me, go to the stage or come for me. He looked like a ball player caught in a pickle between first and second base. At last he made a decision and came back. He walked behind me, his hand on my back to steer me up the steps onto the stage.

I leaned into Aaron and smiled for the camera, pretending the tears in my eyes were tears of laughter—everyone in the room was laughing with us or at us—but in truth my eyes were burning. I kept my head down as we walked off the stage. At the table, Aaron apologized. "I'm such a dork," he said, squeezing my knee. The table buzzed with reassuring comments while I smiled and played good sport.

On the drive home from the awards banquet, Aaron apologized more profusely. "I didn't do it on purpose. I get so frustrated that it's all about money. I just wanted the whole thing to be over."

I squeezed his hand. "I haven't thought any more about it," I said, assuring him it wasn't a big deal. "I won't even remember it next week."

BUT I DID think about it. Constantly. I remembered every day for the next week and long beyond that. With Laiah's help, I rehashed the table scene over and over, analyzing every moment of the evening. Though we didn't doubt Aaron's contrition, we both agreed his act spoke volumes: I had become so insignificant that even dressed to the nines, wearing a black evening dress, sitting right next to him, he entirely forgot I was there.

The problem was I'd said *no* to too many things. I'd declined hosting his client Christmas party and rejected his desire to travel for Christmas. Despite the multiple times a day I cleaned up, the house was usually in disarray when he arrived from work, and he often pitched in and made dinner. Aaron worked so fast he could have the house tidied and dinner ready before I finished my last piano lesson. He made my job look so easy. Most of the time I was so unorganized he had to bail me out. He helped me with my work around the house more than I helped him with his work. He must have thought I hadn't done enough to help him earn the Top Producer Award to merit bringing me to the stage.

There was a time when Aaron admired me, when he thought I was the most amazing woman in the world, but now he viewed me as unspectacular.

I made a decision.

While saying no made life more enjoyable, it wasn't worth it. A person has to be busy and work hard to be recognized, to be worthy of being on stage. I wasn't afraid of hard work. I knew how to stay busy. My mantra needed to change. From then on, no matter how exhausted or stressed I felt, I would say yes to everything. I would travel for Christmas. I would go on weekend campouts. I would do business ideas. I would say yes to anything Aaron suggested. I would say yes to anything people expected of me. I would do anything, *anything*, just so Aaron wouldn't be embarrassed or ashamed to be seen with me, just a housewife.

CHAPTER 11

Yes

Thursday 3:00 p.m.

THE DIGITAL CLOCK on the dashboard shows 3:00. My plan had been to leave home by 10:30 this morning so I would arrive in Tucson with enough time to check into my hotel room and rest before the opening session. House cleaning and loading the car took more time than expected and thus I'm running late, as usual. So despite the contractions, my speedometer has hardly dropped below 80 mph.

Out of nowhere, violent gusts of wind blow across the desert floor and sweep a cloud of sand over the road in front of me. The spray of dirt works its way through the ventilation system and in no time my eyes and throat are filled with dust. Coughing and blinking, I'm driving blind, caught in the middle of a haboob.

I'd never heard of the term haboob until I became an Arizonan. Dry land areas throughout the world—the Sudan, the Arabian Peninsula, and Arizona—are prone to intense dust storms called haboobs. A haboob arrives suddenly, carried on an atmospheric gravity current. It is usually the result of a collapsed thunderstorm in a drought-afflicted land. And isn't that how it goes—the teasing smell of promissory rain in the air collapses into a dry wind, pelting weathered faces with razor-sharp slaps of sand?

In no time the dust fury engulfs my car. The coughing sets off a bout of contractions, each one stronger than the previous, with barely a break between. My abdominal muscles grow tighter, like a leather belt cinching around my organs. I can't see anything. As if being lost and in labor in the desert weren't challenge enough, nature has sent a swirling cloud of doom to compound the situation.

———※———

A FEW WEEKS after returning from the Cloverman awards banquet, my phone rang with the first of what would be a chain of opportunities for me to say yes. It was Brother Stevens from church. "Your name has been submitted as a possible teacher for early-morning seminary this year."

"Yes. Absolutely," I said without hesitation.

I could hear his shock through the receiver. "Don't answer right away," Brother Stevens urged. "I didn't even want to call you. I know you have young children. Teaching seminary is a huge time commitment. It's intellectually and emotionally taxing. Talk it over with your husband. We usually like to give people more notice, so they have months to prepare their lessons plans, but one of our teachers moved unexpectedly."

"Okay, I'll talk it over with Aaron, but I'm ninety-nine percent sure my answer will be yes," I told him.

Seminary is a weekday religion class my church provides for youth ages fourteen to eighteen. The class is taught early morning, before the regular school day begins. This year the seminary curriculum would be the New Testament. I would be an unpaid volunteer teacher—most jobs in my church are unpaid volunteer positions—but I wasn't in it for money. Finding quiet time to study and pray with three kids at home was yet another area in which I was falling short in life. Teaching seminary would force me to make scripture learning a priority.

I told Aaron about the call. "I told him yes."

"You quit the magazine job because it was too much," he responded.

"This will be early in the morning while you're at home. I won't have to buckle kids and drive them to babysitters. I'll be back before they wake up; they won't realize I'm gone."

Aaron looked skeptical.

"Danny starts all-day kindergarten this year. Tanner is easy. I have two free hours to prepare lessons while Kate's at preschool. I need more spirituality in my life."

The whole situation was ideal.

Annice didn't agree. We were sitting on her back patio watching our kids play. "You are going to be so tired." She had taught early-morning seminary when Ashley was young. "It's harder than you imagine."

Hard for some women, I thought, *but I am* not *some women.*

Before the school year began, I prepared object lessons, colored visual aids, and planned learning games. At night I imagined standing in front of my young students leading deep spiritual discussions about the Sermon on the Mount and the Parables of Jesus.

What actually happened the first day of class was that one of the seniors took the paper plate (on which I'd brought home-baked muffins), drew eyes and a mouth, attached a rubber band, and strapped it around his head so he could lean back in his chair and sleep while the eyes on the plate stayed awake. I tried to ignore him and go on with the lesson, but I was spending more time asking students to *stop* talking, *stop* tipping their chairs, and *stop* throwing paper clips than I was teaching about the origin of the New Testament. I had spent hours preparing an amazing lesson, but they only wanted the clock to reach 6:45 a.m. so they could leave. I stormed to the back of the room and grabbed Corbin's plate face, but the elastic twisted in his hair, so as I yanked it out, a tuft of hair came with it. He screamed and grabbed my wrist, we tussled, and I completely lost respect and control of the class.

After a few days, Sister Wardell, the seminary supervisor, phoned me. "Did you know you had students skipping class and coupling off in the janitorial closet? From now on, you need to phone parents if their student doesn't show up for class." From then on, I spent precious lesson preparation time phoning and having long conversations with parents worried about troubled teens.

Annice had been right. So had Brother Stevens. This was harder than I'd expected. At night I couldn't sleep for worrying about my students, my lesson, or sleeping through my alarm. Tanner wasn't happy and self-entertaining with Danny and Kate gone to school. He played fine as long as they were playing nearby. Once home alone, he wanted my constant attention. My hours of expected study time disappeared into family crisis and I never felt prepared enough for each lesson.

And why had I signed up to be the art masterpiece volunteer for Danny's kindergarten class?

One month earlier, I was convinced I needed more in my life. Now I had too much. My schedule was overfull. I could not handle another thing. But my Year of Saying Yes was just beginning.

—◈◈◈—

SO ABSORBED IN seminary pressures, I didn't notice how the Cloverman awards banquet had also left its mark on Aaron. In the months following the table incident—while I was ruminating about how to squeeze more impressive endeavors into my life—Aaron was looking for an exit strategy to leave Cloverman altogether. It took a while for me to clue in. As long as I'd known him, Aaron was always on the hunt for new business opportunities. Usually I listened to his latest brainstorm, nodded at the right places, and anticipated a new idea the next day. So I didn't pay much attention to how Aaron was becoming increasingly restless with work. He made passing comments about how moving people's money from CDs to mutual funds, from bonds to insurance annuities, wasn't stimulating. "I'm not challenged," he'd say. "I get paid a ridiculous amount of money for the little work I do."

At heart Aaron is a builder. He'd built this finance office, started from scratch, labored to get the flywheel turning. Now that the machine was rolling, he didn't feel motivated by the day-to-day repetition of making dollar upon dollar by rolling over IRAs. All day for eight hours he did little else than converse with gray-haired people about facing the end of their life, about death, grief, and trust funds. The job was *old*.

What Aaron wanted was to jump into the real estate market. That fall of 2004, everyone—from the produce man at Safeway, to the garbage man who waved to Tanner every Tuesday morning—had purchased rental properties. Aaron could smell opportunity, but it wasn't in buying high, so where was it? Home prices were climbing so fast people couldn't keep up. Buying and selling properties was the constant conversation around work water coolers, on the playground during moms group, and in the parking lot after church. People questioned why we weren't buying into our share of this cash cow, as if we were fools missing out on the investment opportunity of a lifetime. It nagged at Aaron and he scoured for ways to work the trends in our favor.

While Aaron hadn't figured out how to make the real estate thing work, he had found something else that would. The month of October Aaron didn't talk about his usual thread of twenty different business opportunities. He talked about one: printing. "Bob wants to start a southwest edition of his magazine," Aaron told me one day. "He's looking for help."

"I'm surprised Bob would take me back after I quit on him last year."

"He says you're the best salesperson he's ever had. He asks me every week when you'll be ready to go back to work."

Bob had worked in newspaper and printing since high school. He'd tried to retire three times already, but printer ink ran too strong in his blood. He couldn't give it up, so he was looking for a younger partner who could literally do the leg work of advertising sales. In the evenings Aaron worked numbers, showing me spreadsheets filled with potential revenue sources and streams of residual income from printing. "We could run this magazine in a few hours a week."

What's more, we could run it together. It was our dream. We could work from home. Aaron could have more time with the kids, and I could have less time with the kids. Aaron could wear shorts and T-shirts and I could get out of my sweats, put on real clothes, and interact with adults. As a bonus, the magazine wouldn't print in July and August, since most of the readers were snowbirds. In other words, they left Arizona during the heat of the summer to return to their cooler home states such as Nebraska. Aaron looked at me, giddy with excitement. "We could take the kids north every summer." From the time we'd first arrived in Arizona, during the peak of one of the hottest Julys on record, we had dreamed of being snowbirds ourselves. This magazine would make it possible.

We met with Bob and decided to launch the first issue the next April. Signing my name on the contract made me an official business owner, a legitimate working woman.

Had I known in August, at the beginning of the school year, that by November we would be starting a business, I might not have agreed to become an early-morning seminary teacher. And if I had known, when my pen drew the shape of my name on the business partnership, that I was already several weeks pregnant, perhaps we would have postponed the partnership or the launch of the first issue. But how was I to know that my Year of Saying Yes would extend to the uterine level? While hindsight is 20/20, foresight has never been one of my strong suits.

By November, there were so many outstanding yeses I needed to fulfill, inevitably things were going to collide in a big way. As morning sickness hit, the 4:45 a.m. alarm became my mortal enemy. The first thing I did after arriving at the church building each morning was make sure to set a garbage with a plastic liner at the front of my classroom next to me, just in case.

AT MY FIRST prenatal appointment, Dr. Woods confirmed what the two lines on my drugstore pregnancy test had shown. "You're ready to do this again?"

"Yes." If I smiled every time I thought about being pregnant, maybe the feelings of excitement would eventually follow. I was glad he didn't ask if we'd planned this pregnancy. I felt bad for babies who came into the world on the tail of the words "surprise" uttered for nine months. We had planned to have this baby, we just hadn't necessarily chosen the timing.

Dr. Woods and I discussed my history of preterm labor. "The best thing you can do for this baby is to carry it to full term," he affirmed. "Each baby tends to come faster than the one before." He consulted his gestation calendar and said June 29 was the expected due date, which I'd already calculated. "If you stay off your feet, stay hydrated, and get plenty of rest, you won't need to worry about having a preemie next summer."

I told him about teaching early-morning seminary, about not being able to fall asleep until after midnight while worrying about my lessons and my students, and waking up at 4:30 a.m. I told him that Aaron and I had decided to start a business and how much walking I would be doing to sell ads.

Dr. Woods clicked his tongue. "That is too risky. You need more sleep and to not take on the stress of a startup business." He wrote a prescription to sleep from 10:00 p.m. to 7:00 a.m., to stay off my feet three hours every afternoon, and to eliminate stress. "You have three young children. Add being pregnant to that and your plate is full. Don't add anything else." He made multiple copies of the prescription for me to give to anyone who questioned.

At least, that's what I *wish* had happened.

The truth is I left his office trying to wrap my brain around another pregnancy. Rather than worrying about preterm labor, I was scanning my heart for those tingling feelings of baby excitement. It would come in time. God knows I love babies and would take a baby into my heart and life anytime the heavens wanted to add another child to our family. I had just been caught by...*surprise*.

Thursday 3:05 p.m.

THE HABOOB HOVERS around my car, making it impossible to see the road. When I can't hold on to the steering wheel any longer, my hands grab my stomach trying to guard my womb against the excruciating pressure while my car weaves. There's no choice but to take my foot off the gas pedal, press the brake, and pull off the road. The coughing triggers another round of tightening. I've turned off the air, but can't open the windows to let the dust escape. Being engulfed in gray gloom gives me the sense that I've been swallowed by the storm and now exist in another dimension inside the belly of this beast. I squirm and stretch my back deeper into the seat, hoping the lengthening will create space and prevent my kidneys from being pressed into powder. A terrible whining sound like the siren of an emergency vehicle rises from my throat. *Did I make that noise?* I clamp my mouth shut and hold my breath. The contraction twists and contorts.

It's happening. Anticipating the gush of water that will deluge the front seat, I spread my legs. This is how it feels before the baby drops, right? I rack my memory of previous labors. How did those last hard contractions feel right before the baby crowned? Certainly they weren't harder than these. I don't remember exactly. Once those last hard contractions hit, there's hardly time to think. It happens fast, like a strike of lightning.

This monster contraction begins to release, but another is climaxing before the first recedes, followed by yet another. My head falls into my hands. *This is my fault. I'm so stupid.* I haven't done enough this pregnancy to stay off my feet and slow down preterm labor. How could I possibly have expected to make it forty weeks?

Pressing back into the seat, I squeeze my eyes shut as hard as I can, hunching and dropping my shoulders around the hardness of my stomach, my body trembling.

CHAPTER 12

Magazine

Thursday 3:10 p.m.

AT THIS POINT, I can no longer ask God to make the contractions go away. The best I can hope is for the labor to ease long enough to get to the hospital in Tucson, assuming there is a hospital in Tucson. I was so positive I would make it through the weekend, I didn't even research medical options in Tucson. I'm not worthy of God's help because I quit teaching seminary. It would serve me right to have to deliver my own baby out here under an ocotillo shrub. Instead, I offer a "Lord, let's make a deal" type of prayer. *Please let me make it to the Tucson hospital and I will never quit a church calling again.*

GIVING UP SEMINARY was an agonizing decision. If it had only been me, I could have woken up before 5:00 a.m., sold ads in the morning, taught piano lesson in the afternoon, and dropped off and picked up three children to three different locations in between. It would serve *me* right for having gotten myself tied into that much obligation. But this baby deserved the best chance at a healthy start to life. How could I ever explain to a child that my stupidity caused his or her weak heart and undeveloped lungs?

"I need to quit seminary," I had told Aaron.

"I absolutely agree." He nodded. "You have to focus on taking care of this baby. I'll go to the seminary supervisors and explain the situation."

I *wish* that was how it happened.

What he actually said was "*Why?*"

FOLLOWING OUR WEEKLY teacher's meeting the next Friday, we were standing in the church kitchen helping ourselves to the juice and donut crumbs left by the students. Clearing my throat I said, "I have some news." Everyone stopped chewing and looked at where I'd somehow ended up pinned against the kitchen island. The words spilled out: *I'm a committed person who doesn't believe in letting people down, but…pregnant…bed rest…magazine…* Barely eight weeks along, this announcement broke my cardinal rule to not reveal a pregnancy before fifteen weeks. (My mother rolled her eyes at women who publicized their pregnancy while the sheets were still warm.) "*I'm telling you early so you have the Christmas break to find a replacement.*"

No one spoke for what felt like nine months. They stared, frozen in the literal space of a pregnant pause. And in that parturient silence I didn't look down or hang my head. Rather, I stared back, looking from face to face, noticing mouths hanging open, chins dropped, brows lowered, lips bitten. Was the sink dripping or was it the kitchen clock measuring off seconds? Though no one spoke out loud, I could hear the jumble of words coming at me: *Why would you agree to teach if you were planning to have a baby? Do you realize the bind you've put us in? Where are we going to find a replacement teacher mid-year?*

I seriously considered confessing that although I was *expecting*, this pregnancy was not *expected*, but that would sound like saying this baby wasn't wanted, which wasn't at all true. Wedged into that linoleum-floored serving space, facing three men in dark suits and two women in dresses, I felt a tingle of elation stirring deep in my core. The sensation surfaced from deeper than my stomach or my bones or even my uterus. This sensation—old and familiar—came to me from a remote and proximal place, the location of the origin of my quintessence. The source of my identity—a vast field nourished by the fountain of feminine essence and watered by rains of intuitive nurturing. This sensitivity originated from the very birthplace of *me*, carrying now with it a nervous and delighted anticipation. The words I'd spoken out loud lingered in the air around me. "I am pregnant." These words, or rather, me speaking these words, opened my soul to the wave of sensations—excitement, rapture, the potential of creation—rousing every cell, waking each primal instinct, filling all the levels of me with the marrow of motherhood. *I am carrying a baby.*

Sister Wardell, the supervisor, spoke first. "Well, isn't that great for you." She was not congratulating me. She turned to the tenth-grade teacher, Sister Ostregard. "What are we going to do? I'm leaving next Wednesday for a two-week cruise. My husband and I have been so *busy*, we need to get away. Now I'm going to be stressed the whole time about finding another teacher."

I don't know why she was pointing her dander at Sister Ostregard who had no responsibility for finding new teachers. As the tantrum progressed, Sister Wardell scuffed her feet across the linoleum, huffing, breathing harder with each sentence. The whole scene made me think either she was an angry bull preparing to charge, or she was trying to wipe the vexation of me off her feet onto the kitchen mat. The scene was painful. It would have been easier to keep teaching. At last Brother Stevens intervened. "We are happy for you. We will find a replacement."

Through nausea and fatigue, I taught up to Christmas break, ending my last day of class showing a video about the birth of Jesus and serving holiday treats. All of my visual aids came off the walls and home with me in the trunk of the car. When seminary resumed on the ninth of January, some other woman's chin would be pointed sternly to quiet the class while my chin would be tucked cozy under my bed covers. My heart had felt satisfied that the choice to quit seminary was the best decision for our family.

Until it backfired.

When school let out, we packed what little winter gear we owned and drove north to Utah, pulling the car off the road and letting the kids out to play at the first sight of snow. Helen outfitted my crew with boots, snow pants, and gloves and Grant inflated the snow tubes. Aaron was standing at the top of the sledding hill giving Danny and Kate a push in their shared tube when his cell phone rang. It was Brother Stevens asking if Aaron would take over teaching my seminary class.

And really, how could he say no?

———

ON THE FIRST Wednesday back in Arizona after Christmas break, I heard a knock at the front door. It had to be Bob. Most people rang the doorbell, but Bob was always conscientious that one of the kids might be sleeping, even at 9:00 in the morning. I pulled my hair out of its morning bun, shook it loose, and smoothed it with my fingers. The aftermath of our Christmas was scattered across our front room. The kids had been playing with the boxes and wrapping paper more than with their new toys. After wishing me good morning and asking about our holidays, Bob said, "I'm bringing some things to help you with selling." He pulled out a magazine and showed me the January cover of his northwest edition.

"It looks beautiful. LuDene does an amazing job." My hands flipped through the pages.

"I brought you twenty-five copies and I have a box with a hundred more. We printed extra this month so you could have plenty to hand out."

From October through December, Aaron and I had been playing magazine the way that Danny and Kate play "house." For months we had been setting up our game, now it was time to dig in and get to the business of it. With Bob standing on my front porch handing me business supplies and twenty-five magazines, the sinking reality of the operation fell heavily into my outstretched hands. Bob added a package of dual carbon copy blank contracts on top of the stack of magazines. I felt the work piling up.

Bob described the purpose for each item he handed to me including an alphabetized accordion file for organizing contacts and a set of multicolored highlighters for proofreading the magazine before print. He topped the stack with clear page protectors. "I never give a business owner a plain sheet of paper with their ad proof like other magazines do," Bob explained. "Their proof gets wrinkled or lost on a desk and looks cheap. These protectors show how important their ad is to us and keep it looking professional and valuable."

While I was balancing the box of clear protectors on the stack, Tanner streaked into the living room wearing only a diaper. He charged into me from behind, knocking me forward. Bob reached up to stop me from toppling into him. Tanner wrapped his arms around each of my legs, poked his head through my knees, and grinned at Bob. "Looks like somebody hasn't gotten dressed yet," Bob noted. Was it worth explaining to Bob that I'd already dressed Tanner—*twice?* This was a boy who didn't like keeping clothes on no matter the weather. Tanner dangled on my legs while I tried to casually adjust his weight and pretend he wasn't there. I nodded, encouraging Bob to continue.

Bob pulled out a long, narrow green box. "And you're going to need these." He smiled proudly opening the lid to reveal a long row of white business cards. "They look nice, don't they?" Printed under the Southwest Business Journal logo in red lettering was my name and title: *Maleah Warner, Co-Owner.* In all this process of deciding to start the magazine and create the partnership, I hadn't considered what my title or position would be. Mostly I saw myself deferring to Bob and Aaron and their business experience. But there it was printed in bold, on the first business cards I'd ever had—I owned a magazine.

"And Aaron will need these." Bob pulled out a separate box. The sample card taped to the lid showed the same logo followed by Aaron's name and his position doing layout design.

Danny yelled from the kitchen. "Mom, I can't open the milk."

"Give me just a minute, Danny. I'm busy, then I'll come help you."

"We have just over two months before our first issue..." Bob breathed in a sigh. "We should be able to put out a nice product..." Bob hesitated. "Like I've told Aaron, you're the best salesperson I've ever had." Was he offering that statement to reassure me or him? From the kitchen a series of precarious-sounding *thunks* was followed by a loud crash and the clanking of spilled silverware. Bob looked past me, but I ignored the commotion showing that he needn't worry about my life, my kitchen, or my chaos. *Take heart, Bob, you have my full attention.* By starting this partnership, he was lumping his thirty-year respected newspaper career in with my tilted Christmas tree and broken kitchen drawer.

"One last thing." Bob held up a ream of white paper as if it were his turn for print school show and tell. "This is eighty-pound semi-gloss paper. I never print an ad proof on regular twenty-pound paper because..."

"It looks cheap," we said at the same time.

He smiled and added the ream of paper to my stack.

I held out the package of highlighters like a dangling carrot in front of Tanner. "Take this and put it on Mommy's desk, please?" I asked partly to free up space in my hands, but mostly to get him off my legs. He grabbed the package eagerly, still buzzing with the fresh excitement of Christmas surprises. Only after he'd run down the hallway did I realize that I'd just given a package of markers to a toddler who had spent a lot of time recently learning how to open packaging.

The masked urgency in Bob's voice was contagious. My heart beat with the anxiety of a sprinter who had arrived late to the track and was running to the line before the race had even started. With arms heavy-laden, I said goodbye to Bob and closed the door with my back. I lifted my head to face my Christmas-strewn living room and silverware-scattered kitchen floor, debating whether to begin making a list of potential customers, put away the tree and fix the silverware drawer, or take on my role as the pink power ranger like I'd promised Kate. Tanner ran past chewing on the tip of an orange highlighter and I made a five-yard dash for the office. As a mother, when wondering what task is most important, the answer is simple: Put out the fire that's burning hottest.

———⟊⟊⟊———

THE NEXT MONDAY, January 9, Aaron hit the too-early alarm, groaned, and fell back into his pillow. I waited, wondering if he had fallen to sleep and if I would have to shake his shoulder and say the dreaded words, "You have to get up now or you'll be late." I waited as long as possible, then rolled toward him and placed my hand on his arm.

"I'm awake." He shook off my hand, his voice sleepy and gruff. He took in two deep breaths, each followed by a long exhale, and lifted his body, setting both feet on the floor with reluctance. While Aaron was at seminary, I forced my expanding circumference out of bed and woke Danny with instructions to get dressed for school while I showered. Thus was the beginning of our new routine. While I toweled dry, Aaron came home from seminary and changed from church clothes to business casual. Facing my half of the closet, I scoured the hangers for something to wear that would look professional and also fit around my growing girth. Aaron would drop Danny to school, work a full day at Cloverman, then come home and spend hours teaching himself magazine layout and ad design. After a few weeks, he looked to be in rough shape. "I have no time to prepare a seminary lesson," he would lament. "I totally wing it every day."

My morning task consisted of contacting as many potential business advertisers between 9:00 a.m. and 11:30 a.m., the hours Kate would be at preschool on Mondays, Wednesdays, and Fridays. This would mean waking Kate and Tanner and having the three of us dressed, fed, and ready to buckle in the car by 8:30 a.m. If the morning went well, then at precisely 8:45 a.m. I would knock on the sitter's door with Tanner perched on my hip, and at 8:55 a.m. I would open the car door so Kate could run into Ms. Stacey's preschool. Twenty minutes later I would arrive at my chosen business area in Goodyear, with ninety minutes to convince as many business owners as possible to take a chance at advertising in the *Southwest Business Journal.* Then I would rush to pick up Kate no later than 11:35 a.m. and repeat the process in reverse. Next would be lunch, followed by settling Tanner for an afternoon nap, finding things to engage Kate, and opening the door for my first afternoon piano student. On Tuesdays and Thursdays, Kate and Tanner both spent the morning at the sitter, offering me a full three hours of contacting.

ISN'T IT CURIOUS how you can say yes to something before fully understanding the ramifications? Everything about this business venture had sounded ideal in concept, so I'd signed my name to the endeavor without fully realizing that Aaron wouldn't be doing any of the ad sales. "I'm regulated under FCC law," he explained. "I can't sell anything outside of work or I get shut down."

"When were you going to tell me that?"

"I did tell you. I thought that's why you quit seminary, so you could sell."

I did quit seminary so I could sell, but my brain hadn't processed the fact that the responsibility to win enough advertising contracts to fully fund the printing and mailing costs would rest entirely on me.

On the drive from Ms. Stacey's to Goodyear, I rehearsed my sales pitch. It was one thing to play magazine. It was quite another to persuade business owners to sign a contract agreeing to pay me real dollars every month for the privilege of putting their ad inside my brand-spanking-new publication. Did I sound confident enough, or would they see straight through the facade and recognize I was nothing more than a stay-at-home mother wearing dress slacks and a button-up shirt?

Most of my work was cold contacting, which meant I walked in off the street without an appointment and tried to be friendly enough that the front desk employee would let me speak to the boss. I'd introduce myself and my new magazine. "April will be our first issue and the deadline for advertising is on the seventeenth of March." The pregnancy probably opened more doors than normal. Even cold-hearted people struggle to slam the door in the face of a pregnant woman.

The weekend of our first print deadline, Tanner broke his leg jumping on a trampoline. Aaron took him to the doctor to get his leg x-rayed and casted, then came home and stayed awake until 2:00 a.m. finishing the magazine layout.

Neither Aaron nor I slept well those months. He tossed restlessly worrying about his seminary students, his lesson, and sleeping through his alarm. Even though I was *pregnant* tired, I couldn't nap during the day out of guilt that the dark circles under Aaron's eyes were my fault. If Aaron couldn't nap, I shouldn't either.

As I hit my sixth, then seventh, then eighth month of pregnancy, the balmy March weather became less bearable in April, then turned into May's spiking temperatures. My feet swelled and the arms of my blouses were soaked with sweat. Between business contacts, I sat in the car with the air conditioner blowing full speed to dry out before the next contact. As my weight increased, my equilibrium decreased. One day I teetered off a curb and caught myself on a poor pedestrian who happened to be within my reach. Once the initial morning sickness of the first trimester passed, I grew ravenously hungry and bartered a deal with a Chinese restaurant. They paid for their advertisement in restaurant gift certificates and I fed my growing baby on the number four special: sweet and sour pork with fried rice and an egg roll.

The heavier my belly became, the more I secretly hoped Dr. Woods would put me on limited activity. With Kate I had to stay down and didn't want to; with this baby nothing sounded more appealing than mandatory bed rest. According to new studies—Dr. Woods informed me—it wasn't proven that Brethine was any more effective at slowing contractions than drinking plenty of water and getting off your feet when contractions flare up. So I drank water like an elephant and discovered the locations of the cleanest restrooms in the southwest valley. At each monthly prenatal visit, I held my breath while Dr. Woods monitored my contractions, hoping to hear the words "limit your activity." Instead he would announce, "Everything looks great. This baby is growing right on schedule."

Teaching piano lessons was probably the best thing for the baby, forcing me to sit down every afternoon. Aaron moved the recliner next to the piano in place of the hard kitchen chair I'd been using. Instead of joining my students on the bench for duets or demonstration, my body stayed in that recliner and I called out instructions. On bad days I pulled the lever and kicked out the footrest. From January through May we limped this way through life with bags under our eyes and forgetting essential things, like picking up Danny from school.

CHAPTER 13

Rescue

MY PREGNANCY DREAMS were vivid and bizarre. I began waking from a recurring dream, panting and out of breath. In the dream I was a pregnant cart horse, my hoofs calloused from clomping all day across cobblestone roads in iron shoes, the bulkiness of my body adding weight to the load I pulled. The driver—who had a curly red beard and wore a straw hat—whipped my back relentlessly: "Move, you sluggish beast! No stopping 'til the deliveries are done."

One morning in Goodyear, I was waiting in Ron's Carpet and Tile store when I got dizzy and the room began to spin. *Yes!* I was going to faint right there on the carpet samples and Ron would call for an ambulance. Aaron would arrive at the hospital and rush to my side with a worried expression. The doctor would ask, "What are you doing to this girl?" Aaron would look guilty. The doctor would say, "She has worked herself to the bone. I order a mandatory three-day hospital rest and she must stay off her feet after that." Aaron would actually take a few days off work to watch the kids. Church members would deliver meals. Bob would bring me flowers and say, "Don't you worry one bit about the magazine, young lady. You focus on taking care of yourself and that baby."

But I didn't faint. I went on to sell Ron the perks of being one of the first advertisers in a new magazine. "You lock in the introductory rate and get first choice of the prime locations such as the middle bind. That's where the magazine naturally falls open."

Aaron didn't take time off work. Church ladies didn't bring casseroles. I cooked dinner, mended the rip in Danny's backpack, cut chewing gum out of Kate's hair, treated Tanner for pinworm, collapsed into bed and dreamed the carthorse dream. Only this time, the carthorse looked back but couldn't see the face of the person holding the whip. *Who was driving me so hard?*

What kept me going through all this was knowing it was temporary. If I could build up enough ad revenue in our April, May, and June issues, then Aaron would be able to resign from Cloverman Financial over the summer break. In August he would join me working the magazine full-time.

On May 20, I collected my last ad proof for the June issue. Aaron would layout the magazine tonight and submit it to the printer. He had one week left of teaching seminary and I only had my spring piano recital to finish, then we could breathe for a few weeks before the baby arrived. We were looking forward to our two-month break from printing deadlines.

——⟨∂/∂⟩——

Thursday 3:15 p.m.

THE HABOOB REMAINS, caressing its spindly, gray fingers over the roof and down the hood—a jilted lover saying goodbye, begging to stay one moment longer. I can't stop coughing. It's a bad omen. I should have turned around when I could. God is punishing me for being so foolish. Then, in an eerie dissipation as if milking a final dramatic curtain call, the haboob swirls and condenses into a tight ball, rolls off the hood onto the ground, and breaks apart, releasing a single, trapped tumbleweed which bounces away across the desert floor. Once the dust is gone, I roll down the windows and turn the air to full power. Between coughs, I blow the dirt out of my nose and drink the last sip of water to rinse my throat.

There are no clouds today. Once the haboob clears, the sky reappears as vast and unbroken in its blueness as the land is in its brownness. I'm too nervous to get out of the car and walk around, afraid the standing weight will break my water. Instead, I tilt the driver's seat back as far as it will go, raise the steering wheel and lay back, hoping the change of position will curb the contractions. The interior temperature rises as the car idles. My brothers used to catch grasshoppers and fry their exoskeletons using cub scout magnifying glasses to concentrate the sun's rays into laser beams. The windshield acts as a magnifying glass, scorching my skin; the heat pulls all the water out of me. My throat is dry and parched like the desert ground around me.

With the next contraction I wrap my arms behind the seat and try not to bear down. *Breathe!* My muscles stretch, tightened to capacity. What comes to mind is that ancient torture where soldiers tie four horses to a man's limbs and whack their rumps, sending the horses running in four opposite directions.

Around me the air is ablaze in an incinerator of burning sun. My consciousness goes fuzzy. In the ripple of blurry heat waves, I see the flashing lights of a patrol car spin in the rearview mirror. A shadow darkens my window. The strong hands of a state trooper brush my sticky hair away from my face and firmly press into my neck and wrist checking for a pulse.

"What are you doing out here all alone, pretty lady?" He tsks, and with the back of his hand he feels my forehead. My eyes flutter between open and closed. Ever so gently the palm of his hand feels my enlarged belly; the baby kicks, triggering another contraction. He looks at his wristwatch and counts until the contraction eases up. Without hesitation, but careful not to bump my swollen belly against the steering wheel, he lifts me out of my car. His boot-clad feet crunch the scorching gravel as he carries me back to his squad car and gingerly lays me down—like a delicate porcelain doll—across the back seat. This highway patrol officer sees in me what no one else sees. Everybody thinks I am strong, unbreakable. He can sense what I really am: fragile, like fine china that should be handled with care, taken out for special occasions, not worn-out from daily use.

"Stay with me, sweetheart." His deep voice soothes me. "No pretty ladies or babies lost on my shift." My subconscious submits to his authority. No more worry, he has come to my rescue. My head against the cool leather seat, I sink deeper into unconscious bliss, relinquishing all control, savoring the sweetness of this dream where I don't have to make any decisions because, for a change, somebody else is taking care of me.

———

AARON STOOD IN the door of the student council office one afternoon in mid-March with his arms folded across his chest. "You still owe me dinner." He leaned against the doorframe like I'd better pay up or he wouldn't let me out.

I sat at my desk cramming for a test. "I believe the correct phraseology is that *you* owe *me* a dinner." He had easily lost our bet.

"Oh, I'll buy dinner." Aaron smiled mischievously. "You owe me the presence of your company."

I felt a sneeze coming on and grabbed a tissue from my desk. "Just give me a day and time..." I pressed my nose and stopped the sneeze.

"Wow, you don't sound good." Aaron moved toward me. "Are you sick?"

"My ears plugged up on the flight to debate nationals and they haven't popped since. The whole weekend I could only hear my own voice like a microphone in my head. It's driving me crazy."

Aaron put his hand on my forehead. "You have a fever. Have you seen a doctor?"

"I don't feel that sick. I just wish my ears would pop so I could hear normally."

"You should probably go home and get some rest."

"I can't. I have a Faculty Academic Council meeting at 2:00. President Rawlings wants my report on the possibility of expanding our music program to a four-year degree. Then I tutor microbiology. Tonight is the Dean's List Dinner. I have to pick up helium for the balloons..."

Aaron knelt in front of my desk and looked at my droopy eyes. "You keep going like this and you'll end up taking your impressive resume to an early grave." He closed my textbook and hefted my backpack over his shoulder. "Come on," he coaxed. "A couple hours of sleep will do you good. I'll tell President Rawlings you're sick."

"Jen and Beth's gang will be watching *Days of Our Lives* at my apartment. I won't get any sleep there."

"I have someplace better."

Aaron's room was surprisingly clean and cozy. I had expected posters of red sports cars and super models. Instead, his walls and shelves were covered with family photos and his bed was made.

"Lie down," Aaron ordered, pulling back his comforter. He took off my boots, slid my feet under the covers, then tucked the blanket under my chin. "You are grounded here for two hours."

"I can't miss Dean's List Dinner, Aaron. I'm in charge."

"Don't worry. I'll wake you up. Now sleep."

I fell asleep looking at his pictures: Aaron with a white-haired woman, probably his grandma; Aaron hugging his mom and dad; Aaron wrestling three younger brothers; Aaron petting a brown Labrador.

When I woke up hours later, I yawned, and my ear popped so hard I thought I had burst my eardrum. "Oh my goodness, I can hear!" I wiggled my jaw back and forth and it popped three more times. I felt so much better, but outside the window, the sky was getting darker. What time was it? In front of the clock, I noticed a colorful display that hadn't been there when I went to sleep. There was a can of chicken noodle soup, a bottle of orange juice, a single rose, and a note written in Aaron's handwriting: *Get better, pretty lady*. I dropped back onto the pillow with a satisfied smile. I was not accustomed to receiving this kind of attention.

When Aaron came to get me, he brought my student council shirt to change into and he already had the helium tank in the trunk of his car. "You look good. How are you feeling?" He put his hand on my forehead.

"Thank you for the juice, the flower, the nap…I feel so much better."

He wrapped me in a teddy bear hug. "You deserve it, pretty lady."

———✧✧✧———

Thursday 3:30 p.m.

IT'S THE SILENCE that wakes me. Blinking and focusing, the interior of a car comes into view. The middle console, the air conditioning vents, the buttons to lock and unlock the door. Slowly the realization clears that I'm not lying on the backseat of a patrol car. This is my car. Reaching down, I feel for the lever and raise the driver's seat to the upright position. The clock shows I've been asleep for fifteen minutes. The dream seemed so real.

"Swooning to be rescued?" Laiah laughs when I recount my dream. "We're not drippy teenage girls holding out for the dashing knight and gallant rescue."

She's right, as always. No one forced me to make this trip. Aaron had been adamantly opposed to my coming. Any patrol officer unlucky enough to happen upon me here wouldn't find a delicate damsel in distress. The elastic waistband of my maternity pants has become a water-logged inner tube from catching the drips of perspiration that flowed down my back while I slept. My breasts hang soggy, too wet and heavy for the bra to support any longer. The poor officer would find a sweat-stenched, red-faced blimp who's driven alone into the desert toward a city she's never been before, despite having contractions every five minutes.

I don't deserve to be rescued from the predicament I've created for myself. The tires spin in the gravel before reclaiming their hold on the highway. In the rearview mirror I think I see a brief glimpse of a patrol car and the silhouette of a sturdy officer hunched over a woman, but the image evaporates into the hot air, replaced by nothing but a sterile two-lane highway, stretching for miles in both directions. With the gas pedal pressed to the floor, the car speeds forward while I offer another pleading prayer. *Please, let me make it to the Tucson hospital.*

CHAPTER 14

Tucson

Thursday 3:45 p.m.

IN THE DISTANCE I see multicolored specks and squeal with relief. A few more miles and a scattering of houses and buildings dot the barren landscape. At last a green sign tells me ten miles to Tucson. Now I'm passing sign after sign advertising food, gas, and hotels. Next, the sign I've been watching for appears: A blue vertical rectangle with a white block letter *H* directs which exit will lead to the hospital.

Out the right passenger window, I notice an old, bright orange house on the outskirts of Tucson where a crew of workers are nailing down new shingles on the roof. I know the process well. Last October, during my Year of Saying Yes, we traveled to Utah for fall break. Aaron's parents were in the process of re-shingling their roof. Neither Grant nor Helen asked me to climb the ladder and rip up old shingles with a crowbar, but I didn't want to be left on the ground chasing the kids while Aaron and his brothers had all the fun. Little did I know at the time when I was pounding nails into my in-laws' roof, that another project was under construction inside my womb. Without instruction, cells were forming, dividing, bringing to pass the work of embryonic formation. Growing a human being inside of you is a miraculous thing, but I was oblivious to the miracle last fall when the zygote made its journey down the fallopian tube and settled in my uterus. Even on this, my fourth pregnancy, I'm astonished by the photos in my pregnancy books showcasing the stages of fetal development, from the first division of cells to the beginning thump of the minuscule heartbeat.

My thoughts about the wonder of pregnancy are interrupted suddenly when a worker on the orange house stands and waves his arms frantically. From the motion of his mouth I can nearly hear his warning shouts. A plastic-wrapped package of shingles has been knocked loose and is sliding toward the edge of the roof. The stack hits the ladder which tilts back and rocks slowly. From my vantage point I can only see the roof, but from the way the roofer is yelling, there must be workers on the ground below. The ladder falls, followed by the shingles after it. The roofer slides swiftly to the edge and calls to his coworkers.

This reminds me of a story.

In church growing up there was an oft-repeated lesson that went like this: A man was working on the roof of his two-story house when he lost footing and began to slide toward the edge where he will presumably fall to his death. In fear, the man called out to God, something he had rarely done. "God, please save me. Spare my life and I promise to give up all my vices and to serve you from this day forward." Just as the man reached the edge and was about to plummet to the ground below, his shirt caught on a protruding nail. His fall was interrupted, and the man was able to crawl back onto the roof. Delighted and relieved, the man looked to the sky. "Never mind about all that," he said to God, "I don't need your help after all."

Here is my dilemma.

On one hand, I've been praying for God to help me make it to the Tucson hospital.

On the other hand...for the past twenty minutes I have been trying to visualize delivering this baby in a strange hospital with a strange doctor and my imaginings never end with a pleasant outcome. I don't know anything about Tucson, but my impression is that it's a rustic town, a hardy but well-worn remnant of the old west with horses drinking from a trough in front of the barber shop. The hospital is a dilapidated building with chipping paint, no jetted tubs, no Bose sound systems, and all the doctors are clopping down the halls wearing cowboy boots.

Now, in my life I've known plenty of good men, including my own dad, who wore cowboy boots and could deliver a calf, lamb, or colt. But their methods are different.

I don't want the doctor to break my water using a rusting piece of barbed wire fence.

So I haven't called for Aaron to come. Every time my fingers have traced Aaron's number on my cell phone, I imagine him sitting stiff in a metal chair squished between my gurney and the monitors. He's made the four-hour drive following my tire tracks across the desert to witness the birth of his baby, but about thirty minutes before he arrived, my contractions stopped completely. The graph on the monitor has flatlined. Aaron and I can hardly speak due to the suffocating cloud of tension in the room while we wait for a doctor to release us. I'll want to drive back to Surprise, to Del E. Webb Memorial with their Bose sound systems and jetted tubs and my own Dr. Woods. Aaron will shake his head, bite at the hangnail on his right ring finger, then nod in agreement as the doctor says in his thick country accent, "You can leave and you'll have this baby in the car on the way or I can jab this here piece of wire into you and the baby will be born within the hour."

Aaron will say, "We have a sitter and I drove all this way, let's get the baby here."

At that point, what choice will I have but to let the doctor poke me with his rusty tool?

On top of that, I haven't had a contraction in the last fifteen minutes. The hospital exit is getting closer, but my uterus feels as calm as a china bowl in an apothecary shop. If I don't go to the hospital now, I could make the conference in time to hear most of the keynote address.

This is my proverbial fork in the road. *What should I do?*

One night, this past February, Aaron and I had a fight. We were several weeks into Aaron teaching early-morning seminary and me struggling to find advertisers. We were going to bed late, waking too early, and not sleeping much in between. The print deadline for our first issue was a few weeks away and our eyes were twirling like the red and white spiral the cartoon doctor spins to hypnotize his patient.

"I have to stop teaching piano lessons," I told Aaron.

"Why?" He asked my least favorite question.

Part of me was hoping it would be obvious to him that I should quit trying to juggle piano students on top of everything else. In fact, I'd waited, hoping he would tell me I should quit rather than the other way around. I wanted to hear him say, "You're doing too much. You're working too hard. You've got to take care of yourself and the baby."

Instead, I had to explain. "I'm not quitting for *me*. I *want* to teach piano lessons, but if I overdo things now and have to go on bed rest, what would happen to the magazine?" I was the benevolent one here, giving up my piano lessons for the sake of our business.

In a voice fueled by stress and exhaustion, Aaron spurted out, "Sure. Why don't you quit piano just like you quit seminary? Just like you quit *everything*!"

The comment hit a nerve. Before I knew, my hand had struck him hard across the face. He reached up and touched the stinging red print of my palm on his cheek. Both of us stepped back, scared to have stirred up the previously untouched potential that existed to physically harm the other. The bruise on Aaron's cheek faded, but I carried the mark—like a cattle brand—that Aaron viewed me as a quitter. When I told Laiah about the fight, she reminded me that comments spoken in sarcasm and anger carry the most truth. I continued to teach piano.

I'VE BEEN SENT two signs: a blue hospital sign and a calm uterus.

Which sign is from God?

No matter how hard I try to visualize a happy, joyous birth experience at the Tucson hospital, the image always ends with me strapped to stained sheets flatlining on the monitors while Aaron, angry and annoyed, peels chipped yellow paint off the walls.

Ignoring the hospital exit, I stare ahead and continue straight into the city. I've made it this far and I'm no quitter. The only way I'll end up at the Tucson hospital this weekend is if someone carries me there on a stretcher.

⸻ ❧ ⸻

THE ACTUAL CITY of Tucson is different from what I expected. I expected Old Town as in saloon and Wells Fargo Wagon. Instead, it's just old. Old buildings, old stores, old roads. I think I know my way to the hotel, but get turned around and end up in a questionable part of town before at last pulling into the parking lot of the Best Western.

The registration line stretches down the hall. A voice from the conference room introduces the guest speaker. I skip the line and head for the bathroom to relieve my bladder. I dab my sweaty armpits with paper towels, splash water on my face, and wipe away black mascara smears. My face looks like I've been through six rounds in a boxing ring. After refilling my water bottle at the drinking fountain, instead of getting in the back of the long registration line, I walk directly to the conference room. A host is checking the name badges of people waiting to enter. With a pat on my belly, I signal to the host that I'd left my name badge on my seat due to a pregnancy-induced bathroom emergency. The host smiles and nods me inside. There are perks to pregnancy. Perhaps a pregnant woman couldn't get away with murder, but she can get away with entering a conference without a name badge. I'll sign in later once the line has diminished. I don't want to miss the keynote.

On stage, Jane McGrath is teaching how to motivate practicing by selecting exciting repertoire. Spotting an empty chair on an outside aisle, I take the notebook and pen from my shoulder bag and copy down her suggested music for each level. The lights go dark. On the screen appears video examples of Jane's students and approaches she used to address their varying abilities. In my chair I hunker over my notebook and breathe through contractions. When the contractions get too hard, I stand against the wall. Over the course of the opening session I go to the bathroom and refill my water bottle three times, trying to drown out the labor. During one break I phone Aaron quickly to let him know I made it. "How are you doing?" he asks.

"Fine. The conference has already been really good. I'm so glad I came. Better go, they're starting again."

That evening there is a welcome dinner, which I didn't pay to attend. The other teachers leave to mingle in the banquet room. By the time I walk away from the front desk holding my room key, the thought of soaking in the hotel jacuzzi sounds divine, but vanity prevented me from packing my old, stretched swimsuit. A hot bath in my room will have to suffice. The key card buzzes, the door clicks, I switch on the light and enter my hotel room. There is no tub, only a shower.

Once I finish my dinner of carrot sticks and a tuna fish sandwich, I change into pajamas and place my shoes and clothes on the nightstand in case I have to make a fast dash to the hospital in the night. Propping all two pillows against the headboard, I climb into the covers, relieved at last to be off my feet. My body feels like it's been through a full day of consecutive heavy-duty spin cycles.

Listening to the voices of other hotel guests walk outside my door, I stare through the window and think about the day. It is stretching my luck to the point of snapping to think this baby can make it another three weeks. Throughout this pregnancy I have not stayed off my feet. The past nine months of my life has been flooded by a torrential downpour of non-restful activities. Stretching my legs under the sheets, I can still feel the muscles I pulled last August when we cleaned out my parents' house. I don't want to remember anything about that weekend, but before my mind can shut down for sleep, it has to relive the experience one more time.

A WEEK INTO teaching seminary, my brother Paul called with news that my parents had sold our childhood home while they were living in Phnom Penh, Cambodia, as missionaries. "The closing is in two weeks. We're all meeting at the house next weekend to put everything in storage."

According to my mantra for the year, I said, "Yes. Of course I'll be there."

The news meant another bet I'd lost to Aaron. I'd bet him my inheritance that my dad would never sell his farm. Growing up, I was amazed by the so-called army brats who had moved eight times and been to six different schools by the seventh grade. Me? I'd lived in the same state, town, and pink brick house all of my life. Until I'd left for college, the farthest I'd ever moved was from the upstairs shared girls' room to a basement bedroom of my own.

When we gathered in the driveway of our childhood home, we looked to be a motley crew of moving misfits. Most of us were unfit to be moving anything more than our pinky finger. Paul had been twenty-four hours without sleep after covering a hectic ER shift. My younger brother Vern was recovering from having thirty-six inches of intestine removed after a botched colonoscopy. Paul's wife was almost nine months pregnant with their fourth baby. My oldest brother, Karl, with his history of hernias and back issues, would be coming with our youngest brother the next day. The rest of the crew consisted of an assortment of sisters-in-law and a smattering of young nieces and nephews.

My sisters-in-law volunteered to work in the fruit room, boxing the bottled preserves where they could also keep an eye on their babies. Paul said, "Dad and Mom asked that Vern not lift anything. They don't want Karl or Maleah or Deedee to lift anything either."

"So, who is going to lift all this?" I asked. We were looking at six rooms loaded with furniture, three full storage rooms, a wall of bookcases, a cedar closet packed with clothes covering the decades, four full-size metal filing cabinets, two metal safes, an entertainment center, and who knows how many fifty-pound buckets of wheat, rice, oatmeal, and honey. And that was only the basement. We hadn't yet opened the doors to discover what was stacked in the garage, the mudroom, or the outer shed. "Who is going to lift all this?" I repeated.

Undaunted, my eleven-year-old nephew stepped forward. "I can."

"Okay Benji, you're with me," I said.

"The furniture and non-perishable stuff are going into the barn. All the food is going into the horse trailer and back to my house," Paul instructed.

For two days Benji helped me heft beds, bookcases, dressers, and boxes of bottled fruit up the basement stairs and into a horse trailer. I don't remember eating lunch. I don't remember going to the bathroom. I do remember the feel of my T-shirt pasted to my back with perspiration and the red bandanna tied around my head, soggy and dripping sweat into my eyes. After the first day, we pulled the horse trailer over the mountain canyon to Paul's house, where we unloaded everything we'd just loaded, and carried it down his basement stairs to be stacked in piles in his storage room. Paul's wife set out bottles of pain killer along with soup she'd made for dinner. The next morning we drove over the mountain to fill another load.

Sunday night after my flight back to Arizona, I set my alarm for 4:45 a.m. and fell into bed wishing I had thought to arrange for a seminary substitute. When the alarm rang, my muscles were stiff and sore—like the rusty Tin Man from *The Wizard of Oz*. I limped for weeks, my legs and back screaming in pain.

A few months later I signed a contract to start a magazine and took a pregnancy test.

It seems I haven't stopped since.

———*∿∿∿*———

Friday 9:00 a.m.

WHEN THE SUN lights up the hotel room, it takes me a moment to remember why I'm in a hotel bed. Relieved to have made it through the night, I shower and eat my sack breakfast, pleasantly surprised to be feeling much better. No abdominal tug-of-war so far this morning.

My first breakout session begins with a Yamaha dealer showing off his new line of digital pianos and portable keyboards. The next session is on the opposite corner of the hotel property. I traipse the distance in flimsy sandals wishing for better shoes. The walking riles up a few contractions and I spend the class standing in the back listening to ideas for group theory lessons. When class ends, I follow the crowd to the general session.

On Saturday, I'm happy to have lasted another night in the hotel. During the lunch break, I visit the conference music store and purchase two years' worth of music for each of my students. With the individual lesson plans I've outlined for each student, I'm convinced that when I resume teaching in August, they will be every bit as enthusiastic as I am about the hours and hours they will want to practice. After the closing speaker, I pack my suitcase in the car and leave Tucson. The farther away I drive from its hospital, from the exit sign, from the newly-shingled orange house, the more relief I feel. On the drive, there are no desert mirages of coyotes and a sand-covered baby. I'm not actively contracting, but if my water suddenly broke, I would speed, or call an ambulance, which would surely deliver me to the doorstep of Del E. Webb Memorial Hospital and to the gentle hands of Dr. Woods.

CHAPTER 15

Short Kiss, Long Look

Saturday 5:00 p.m.

SATURDAY EVENING, I pull into the driveway of my house, turn off the ignition, and sit.

I made it.

When Aaron opens the front door, I give him a short kiss and a long look. We had each placed a bet on the outcome of this weekend and my look lets him know I had won. Danny, Kate, and Tanner buzz around me like a swarm of bees and I walk to the kitchen dragging my legs under their weight. The house is spotless—all the laundry clean, folded, and put away. Aaron has made dinner: steak and foil-wrapped salmon on the barbecue with corn on the cob and skillet potatoes.

"How were your contractions while you were in Tucson?" he asks while we eat.

"No different than usual." My look says *I told you I wouldn't have this baby in Tucson. You should never doubt me.* Conveniently, I fail to mention the scorpions or the vultures pecking at the dried carcass. "Anybody else want to swim in the jacuzzi tonight?" The kids stand on their chairs and jump up and down cheering, except for Tanner, who is strapped into his booster seat. After dinner we strip the kids down to their skivvies and sit in patio chairs watching them run across the grass with cherry popsicle juice dripping down their bare torsos.

"Have you decided on a name?" I hit the baby ball back to Aaron's side of the court. Our solution to settling the disagreement about whether to find out the baby's gender was that I closed my eyes during the ultrasound while he looked. Thus, he came to have the assignment of choosing the baby's name. From the bedroom he brings out a scrap piece of paper where he's handwritten his ideas. In one column there are a dozen names for boys. In the other column there are only two girl names which look like they'd been hastily added on his way out of the bedroom. Now I also know the baby's gender. Kate will *not* be getting a little sister. "I like the name Jack."

Once the kids are tucked in for the night, I wriggle into my bathing suit. My mirror reflection looks like the Purple People Eater has swallowed a watermelon. Tiptoeing across the cement patio, I climb the wooden stairs and sink into the tepid water like a bloated submarine. "Ahhh, that feels good." The jets massage the overworked muscles in my lower back. The buoyancy of the water lifts the weight of my belly, and I float to the surface. With the magazine deadline, my spring piano recital, the ASMTA conference behind me, and the kids headed into their last week of school, my mind is free to outline my next to-do list. Leaning back and studying the stars, I work out my summer calendar.

There is a joke in my family that if I'm assigned to bring dessert to a party, I will put the cake—which takes thirty-five minutes to bake—into the oven fifteen minutes before the party is scheduled to begin. Stretching resources to last beyond their natural capacity is a quest for me, whether it's nickels, toothpaste, or a pound of hamburger. But you can't cheat time. All these months of planning and calculating, I have failed to finish working the math problem. If I am indeed pregnant a full forty weeks, then this baby won't be born until three days before the Cloverman Financial Family Summer Retreat and won't even be two weeks old for his baby blessing, which is scheduled for the Sunday after Aaron's brother's wedding.

I quickly stand and get out of the jacuzzi realizing that, at this point, I don't want to slow the contractions. Suddenly, hitting forty weeks isn't as important to me as having a baby who is adjusted to breastfeeding *before* we pack up and leave home. In fact, the sooner the baby comes, the better.

In the house I rinse off with a cold shower and crawl into bed where I mentally scan June's calendar and devise the ultimate childbirth scenario.

Tomorrow is Sunday and I play the organ for church. (My aunt's water broke while playing the organ for church. With great composure, she finished the closing hymn before waddling out to her car to head for the hospital. But I don't want that to happen.)

There is an open slot on Monday morning ideal for delivery. I'll wake up early, clean the house, do laundry, stock the refrigerator, and bring my hospital bag to my OB appointment at 10:30 a.m. Dr. Woods will check my contractions and immediately admit me to labor and delivery. I'll deliver a healthy baby, share the glittering birth moment with Aaron, teach the baby to breastfeed without a glitch, introduce the baby to Danny, Kate, and Tanner, chat with visiting family and friends, and eat hospital food. Tuesday I will wake up, pass all tests, and check out of the hospital. I've already calculated that no epidural and a twenty-four-hour hospital stay will save us $1,500. Tuesday I'll bring baby home, welcome the kind Samaritan who delivers hot dinner, and sleep in my own bed.

Then, on Wednesday, all six of us will go to Danny's kindergarten graduation.

It's the perfect plan.

———✦———

Monday 10:30 a.m.

MONDAY MORNING I wash my hair, shave, rub lotion everywhere, and put on makeup. Despite tipping the scale to the heaviest weight of my life, today I feel considerably light. The only thing bothering me is that since Saturday, I've only had a few sporadic contractions. That will change after I've grocery shopped, washed my laundry, and packed for the hospital.

At Dr. Woods' office the nurse escorts me to a room and starts to close the door without handing me a gown. "Isn't Dr. Woods going to check me today?" I ask in dismay.

"Let's see, how far along are you. You are almost thirty-seven weeks…"

"Almost thirty-eight weeks. I ovulate early."

"Have you been having contractions?"

"Yes. I had a lot over the weekend." I don't mention that when I woke up this morning, my uterus stayed sound asleep, exhausted from the ordeal it put me through over the weekend. Though I've lifted gallons of groceries into my car and done everything imaginable to overexert this morning, my uterus is still not contracting. But no need for the nurse to know all this.

"Do you want him to check you?" she asks.

"YES! I mean, yeah, I think he probably should. I usually deliver early and fast."

"Okay." She opens a cupboard and hands me a paper skirt to wrap around my waist.

"Hello!" Dr. Woods breezes cheerfully into the room. He is the nicest, most gentle man. Rumors are he is gay, which causes me to wonder why he chose an occupation focused on female anatomy. I don't know if the rumors are true, but the thought makes me feel less uncomfortable when he sees me naked. "How was your weekend?"

The words come pouring out of me—the four-hour drive, the scorching sun, the sweat dripping between my breasts, the raging contractions, the vultures. The nurse didn't need to know any of this, but I need Dr. Woods to know every detail. "I thought I might have to check in to the hospital in Tucson, but I didn't. I was brave. I toughed it out because I want *you* to deliver this baby."

He laughs but says, "Be careful not to wait too long. Over the weekend we had a mother deliver in the parking lot. I wasn't on call"—Dr. Woods shakes his head—"but Dr. Black said she was ten feet from the entrance."

I try to imagine...

"Let's see if those contractions did anything." Dr. Woods helps me lie down and guides my feet into the stirrups. After a bit of reaching he says, "Oh. Wow."

That's a good sign.

He feels around a little more just to be sure. "Yep. You are fully effaced and really soft. I'd say you are a six." A six! That's better than I'd hoped. He would never let me walk out of here dilated to a six. "Are you having contractions right now?" Dr. Woods asks.

"I had a few this morning."

"Have you had any since you've been in the office?" he asks.

"Well, no," I admit.

"They have me triple booked today. I have forty scheduled appointments." Dr. Woods sounds truly apologetic. "I can't admit you to labor and delivery unless you are actively contracting." In other words, he can't justify rescheduling appointments to deliver anyone who isn't strangling his neck and screaming to push. "By checking you I probably stirred things up enough that you'll be in on your own this afternoon," he offers.

He pats my shoulder in sympathy and closes the door, leaving me half-naked on the table, feeling dejected and wanting. I throw the paper skirt in the trash and pull my maternity pants over my belly button, which closely resembles the cavernous span of the Grand Canyon. "Why couldn't you have behaved like this on Thursday?" I question the bulge. At the checkout desk the secretary schedules me another routine appointment for the next Monday.

"Can I find out which doctors are on call at the hospital outside of regular office hours?" I don't want a repeat surprise appearance from Dr. Babich. The secretary tells me Dr. Woods is on call tonight and again on Wednesday. Like he said, he probably stirred things up enough that I'll be back in a few hours. If this baby doesn't come today, then it needs to wait until after graduation on Wednesday. I try to process the reality that Danny is graduating from kindergarten when it seems so recently that I was going to the hospital to meet him for the first time.

⸻ ⁀⁀⁀ ⸻

Tuesday 8:00 a.m.

TUESDAY MORNING I'M still as round as a bowl of jelly. Expecting to be in the hospital, I have no idea what to do with my day of limbo. The kids need new summer clothes, but I'm sore and cramping from yesterday's exam. I lack the energy and motivation to drag the kids through a series of stores, plus, I'm afraid of my water breaking: *Cleanup on aisle seven*. Besides, Dr. Woods isn't on call, and I don't want to chance missing Danny's graduation, so I try to stay off my feet. After dinner, Aaron sets his plate in the sink and kisses my forehead. "I'll keep my cell phone turned on vibrate," he says as he leaves for his weekly church meeting. I have been contracting all day, but at this point these contractions are going to have to wait until tomorrow. If I'm still contracting like this after Danny's graduation, I'll go to the hospital and check myself into labor and delivery when Dr. Woods will be on call again.

The minute Aaron leaves, the kids turn into wild banshees. I rest my head on the table. "Eat your noodles, Tanner," I say. "Danny, sit down in your chair until you are all the way finished. You cannot run laps around the table between bites." While I clean up dinner, the kids climb from the kitchen chairs onto the half wall and dive bomb into our gigantic bean bag. "No more jumping for the rest of the night," I order while I move them away to scrub sticky handprints off the wall where they've been climbing. "Who wants a story?"

"Me, me, me." They scoot the kitchen chairs over to the bookshelf and begin pulling out piles of books.

"Whoa," I say, catching a stack of books mid-fall. "If you will be very good, take a quick bath, and help me get your pajamas on, I will read you three stories. You can each choose one." I don't know how I will manage kneeling on the tile and leaning over a tub trying to scrub slippery, splashing kids, but I want everyone to be clean for graduation. Danny, especially, needs to be polished and shiny for his big day.

After baths, we pile onto my bed, but the bribery doesn't settle them down like I'd hoped. Their spring is springier than ever as they jump on the mattress. "No jumping, or we won't read, and you'll go right to bed," I say. They lay down on each side of me and I open the first book.

Partway through *Green Eggs and Ham*, a knee-bending contraction takes my breath. I fold myself in half, wincing in pain.

"Keep reading, Mommy," three voices chime.

When the contraction eases, I open the book and resume where I left off. "I would not, could not in a boat, I would not, could not with a g-oooooohhhhhh-oat." I can't help but writhe on the bed, arching my back. Instinctively I grab for Tanner and hold on for dear life.

"Ouch." Tanner pushes my arm and tries to wriggle free.

With a pause in the story, Danny and Kate resume jumping on the bed. I roll over just in time to miss Danny landing his knees in my stomach. "Guys, we'll have to finish the rest another time," I say, panting. I shoo them off the bed, telling them it's late and the bedtime monster will be checking soon to see who is sleeping. "He doesn't eat sleeping children. He only likes that taste of children who are still awake after bedtime." I lock the bedroom doors and begin to pace the hallway, debating whether or not to call Aaron's cell phone.

I made it through Tucson, I remind myself. *I can tough it out one more night.*

CHAPTER 16

Jack

Tuesday 10:00 p.m.

AARON RETURNS FROM his church meeting later than usual and slides into bed next to me. In no time he's breathing deeply. Meanwhile, the war raging in my uterus keeps me wide awake. After midnight I give up on the bed and pace the hall before sliding open the back door and sit in the swing for reprieve. Ten more hours until kindergarten graduation. This is exactly where I was with Tanner two years earlier: sitting in a swing, contractions raging at a fever pitch after midnight. That time I caved, woke Aaron, and went to the hospital. But one hour in the hospital's jetted tub and those roaring contractions were mellow as a kitten. No way I'm caving in tonight.

I can do this.

Deciding to try the hot bath technique, I fill the tub with clean water. While the faucet runs I go to the medicine cabinet and swallow two Tylenol PM pills, hoping they will take the edge off the pain and help me fall asleep. Sinking neck deep, the water pools and recedes over my stretched belly. This isn't the large jetted tub like the one at the hospital with Tanner; still I breathe deeply using a cloth to rub the contractions away. The Tylenol PM kicks in and suddenly my eyes won't stay open. I want to climb back into cozy pajamas, curl in bed, and sleep for days. Instead the muscles tighten under my hands, forcing me to sit forward and grip the edge of the tub. Transferring to my knees, I hold the tub and try to stand, but another contraction knocks me down. As I hunch over, puffing short breaths, my hands reach for the wall, leaving wet prints on the cloth shower curtain and the floral wall paper. There is a shooting pain. My knees buckle and I fall against the wall catching myself on the towel rack.

Then a pause during which I towel dry and step into my sweat pants.

Wednesday 1:07 a.m.

Six hours until the hospital shift changes and Dr. Woods will be on call. If I can't make graduation, at least let the baby hold on until 7:00 a.m. *Come on, uterus. You made it through Tucson, you can make it through the night.*

The pacing resumes; I cover the distance from the front to back door like a swimmer doing laps. The contraction that hits as I pass the kitchen table stops me in my tracks, paralyzing me with the pulling. The umbrella opens. Behind my squeezed-shut eyes is the image of a woman squatting over the blacktop in the hospital parking lot. I crawl on the tile, then grope the wall for support, making my way back to the bedroom. Cowering on the floor next to Aaron's side of the bed, I reach up and shake his shoulder. "Aaron, we've got to go." He looks peaceful. I'm the midnight burglar again breaking in to rob his night's rest. I shake harder. "Aaron." I nearly roll him off the bed. "We better go or you might be delivering this baby at home."

"How long have you been awake?"

"I never went to sleep."

"You didn't? What have you been doing?" Aaron sits up looking alarmed and caught off-guard.

"I took a Tylenol PM and a bath, so now I'm really sleepy. Can you call Patsy to stay with the kids?"

At the intersection of Reems Road and Grand Avenue, Aaron slows for the red light. "Don't stop!" I shout, gripping the door handle and squeezing my legs together. He scans for oncoming cars and runs the light.

Wednesday 2:45 a.m.

After that, everything blurs like a European bullet train. The clock in the hospital lobby shows 2:45 a.m. as the elevator doors close, then reopen to Labor and Delivery triage. One look at my face and the nurse whisks us into a room, stuffing a gown into my chest. While I'm changing in the bathroom, the umbrella in the pelvis opens wider. The sound of my voice echoes back to me, something about "help" and "baby's head." The door opens. Aaron and a nurse catch me, scoop me up, and cart me onto a delivery bed.

There's a gloved finger. "She's a ten plus! Call the doctor!"

Suddenly I'm the unit's main attraction. Two nurses collide, sending trays of instruments flying. A medical student sporting a wild case of bed head shuffles in, stretching and rubbing his eyes looking as if he's been awakened from his comfy roost in an unused supply closet. Every bored graveyard-shift worker has arrived to help set up the room. One by one a crowd forms a semi-circle around me. The nurses stand at the door with a surgical gown and gloves stretched out, waiting for the real star to arrive.

At last he appears in the doorway, moping drowsily into the gown and gloves as if he's sleepwalking.

It's Dr. Babich.

I don't have time to ask if he's washed his hands.

He doesn't have time to say, "Push!"

I sneeze.

Dr. Babich barely lifts his hands in time to catch the slippery ball of baby. He raises his arms like he's holding up the Doctor of the Year trophy.

A strapping baby boy.

Aaron cuts the cord. The nurse lays my boy, slimy and naked, on my chest. "Hello baby Jack," I whisper. He cries intermittently and tries to open his eyes beneath all the goop on his skin. He looks more alien than human, but it doesn't matter. I am hooked. A force flows through me—perhaps instinct, perhaps intuition, perhaps love, most likely a combination of all three. In this moment I know I will do things I didn't know I was capable of doing to any person or any thing that attempts to harm him. I've just now met him for the first time; still, I know my life and heart will never be the same.

The nurse lifts Jack away and takes him to the incubator for measurements. From the bed, with my feet still propped in the stirrups, I anticipate his weight like an Olympic skater watches for her judges' scores.

Seven pounds, one ounce!

I broke my personal record and delivered a seven-pound baby! The mothering judges better give me credit for going thirty-eight weeks—my longest pregnancy—and bonus points for not having an epidural.

But, did I have an episiotomy?

"Ouch!" Searing pain shoots through me from the bottom up. *What is going on down there?*

"Sorry, could you feel that?" Dr. Babich pulls my focus away from Jack's exam on the far side of the room back to where he is still crouched between my spread-open legs.

"What are you doing?" I thought we were all done down there.

"Stitching your episiotomy."

Is it my imagination or is there a 3:00 a.m. look of vengeance in his eyes?

And that's how I discover the one thing in the world that could possibly be more painful than natural childbirth: the stitching of an episiotomy without an epidural.

"I'll get some lidocaine. Usually women are numb enough from childbirth they don't feel anything there for a while."

Those women sound highly *unusual* to me. Dr. Babich gets a syringe and injects lidocaine around *the area*.

Poke. *Yes, I felt that.*

Poke. *And that.*

Dr. Babich makes a dozen injections and I feel every single one. The lidocaine offers a little numbing, but my nerves are acute enough to discern a double cross-stitch pattern. *Is he stitching a replica of the Eiffel Tower?*

He pushes back the wheeled stool and admires his work. Standing and removing his gloves, he reaches into a pocket and pops two-month-old Easter candy in his mouth as he says, "Congratulations." Which I think translates as, *If I ever see you in this hospital again on a holiday or between the hours of midnight and 4:00 a.m., you're going to get a lot worse than the Eiffel Tower.*

I say, "Thank you." Which translates as, *What are you whining about? You're getting good money for a football catch and some crooked needlepoint.*

It turns out that Dr. Babich also broke a record tonight. He scored his personal best for longest episiotomy.

"DO YOU WANT to hold him?" Aaron hands me a tightly swaddled, blue-striped cocoon. My hands unfold the blanket and examine our son closely from his conehead to his tiny feet. He is long and leggy, like my dad. Minutes earlier—balled into the fetal position and squashed inside of me—he had been more the *concept* of a baby, the *possibility* of a person than an actual human. Now he is here and I can't imagine how I ever existed in life without him.

Jack looks around taking in his surroundings. He puts his little hand in his mouth and sucks. Without asking permission, the nurse pulls my hospital gown aside and stuffs Jack's head hard into my chest. *Watch out, lady, I have done this three times before.*

A different nurse wheels an IV cart into the room. "Are you right- or left-handed?"

"Right-handed." My fingers stroke Jack's forehead while he suckles. "Why?"

"I'll put your IV in your left hand." She uncoils clear plastic tubing and rips the sterile wrap off a large needle.

"I don't need an IV."

"It's the best way to administer the Pitocin," she explains.

Did you get your nursing license from a Cracker Jack box? Can you see the baby I'm holding? "I already delivered," I say simply.

"The Pitocin helps with the afterbirth and shrinks the uterus."

My fingers stop caressing Jack's soft face. *How can I escape crazy nurse?* The reward for natural childbirth is *not* having a two-inch needle jammed into the back of my hand. I want my prize! "Oh, no thank you. I wouldn't care for any Pitocin today," I tell the nurse politely, as if she's a waitress who's asked if I want more salt with my food. "I have a good uterus that shrinks on its own."

The nurse glares.

Apparently...hospitals have policies.

Shifting Jack I let her access my left arm. She'd better not say one thing about my perfect veins. She attaches the tubing with a generous amount of tape pressed securely to the hairs of my arm. I'll need an epidural to get the tape off. The IV ties me to the bed; my left arm becomes useless. The cool liquid flows through my veins and in no time I am shaking like kernels in a popcorn machine.

As quickly as all the nurses and doctors had spun into the room to get ready for the delivery, they gather their tools and disappear, like pushing rewind on a VCR and watching the movie backward. The last one out of the room turns off the light and closes the door, leaving Aaron and me sitting in the dark.

"Do you want to hold him?" My voice quivers.

"Are you okay?" Aaron asks.

"I'm shaking so much. I'm afraid I'll drop him."

Aaron re-swaddles Jack, who has been jarred loose from his blanket by my trembling arms.

"What time is it?"

Aaron scans the room for a clock. "It's about 3:30 a.m."

Time and space are distorted. A few hours ago I was home trying to fall asleep. Then a whirlwind. Everyone buzzing, spinning, shouting "Ten plus!" The pain. Oh my gosh, the pain! The burning. The intense need for everything to come out.

"Hey, are you okay?" Aaron asks again.

There is a disconnect between me and my voice, it requires all my effort to form words. "I'm…s-s-so…c-c-cold." Mini-earthquakes erupt simultaneously in various regions of my anatomy. The tremors escalate until I can't tell if I am rattling the bed or if the bed is rattling me. "Aren't…y-y-you…c-c-cold?" I ask Aaron.

"It's June. It's over a hundred degrees outside."

The temperature between the bed sheets plummets to subzero levels. My blood freezes inside the veins. The shaking threatens to bounce me off the bed where I will shatter like frozen glass upon hitting the floor. A blurry image of Aaron carrying the cocoon to the door and light in the hallway. Is he leaving me here to congeal into ice?

"Can we get some help? My wife is freezing and she can't stop shaking."

A nurse brings a thin, overly-washed hospital blanket. "The adrenaline. It's normal. The shaking will go away gradually."

While I huddle and convulse under the blankets, Aaron holds Jack. We both drift in and out of restless sleep. About 6:00 a.m. he nudges my shoulder. "I'd better go relieve Patsy. Are you okay?" I nod. I'm finally warm. With no one around except me and my new baby, asleep in the hospital crib next to me, I drift into deep, deep sleep.

Book Two

Bringing Home Baby

CHAPTER 17

Graduation

Wednesday 7:00 a.m.

"KNOCK, KNOCK?" A head pokes through the door to my hospital room letting in a column of light from the hallway. "You couldn't wait a few more hours for me?" the voice jokes. The voice is familiar, but through the fog of sleep, I can't place the owner. It's impossible to tell if I've been asleep for five minutes or five hours. "Well, I don't want to disturb you." Offering a politely whispered congratulations, the voice retreats and closes the door, returning the room to darkness.

"No, don't go! Come in." Too late I realize the voice belongs to *my* doctor, Dr. Woods.

Sitting up, my bearings finally come to me along with a desperate urge to talk to him. It must be 7:00 in the morning and Dr. Woods is on-call and making his rounds. He needs to know what happened! He's been reading this book with me for nine months; doesn't he want to know how it ends? Of course he can check my chart or speak to Dr. Babich, but I need him to know *my* story. He needs to know about the Tylenol and the bath, the way I marked laps around my house trying to get through the night. Propping up on the hospital pillow, the thought that plagues me is if Dr. Woods perceives me as an adulteress who, in a moment of weakness, sneaked off to another doctor in the night.

The sunlight through the window rises with layers of regret. Four hours! If I could have held on four more hours, then I wouldn't have disturbed the sleep of Aaron, Patsy, and the poor intern. Dr. Babich wouldn't regard me as "that one annoying lady." Dr. Woods would have delivered and my pudenda wouldn't be sewn together by a crooked river of stitches. Will Dr. Woods have to split his commission because I couldn't hold on four hours?

Fully awake, I press the call button and ask for my IV to be removed so I can shower. No one else will catch me groggy and off-guard. Today is a big day! There is a new Warner baby *and* my oldest son graduates from kindergarten.

My hair is washed and blown dry, my lips colored red, and my lashes darkened with mascara when I come out of the bathroom and sit in the guest chair to put on my shoes. A cafeteria worker delivers a breakfast tray and mistakes me for a visitor. "Is the mother in the bathroom?"

"I am the mother."

A new nurse comes to check my vitals. While she tightens the blood pressure sleeve, I ask her opinion. Does she think it's best to bring Jack with me to the graduation or let him sleep in the nursery? Her forehead crinkles in a look that asks if I've just stepped out of an alien spaceship. "You can't leave the hospital without being released."

That makes no sense. Last night I brought myself in voluntarily; I'm not a hospital prisoner. "The school is practically right across the street." *She'll come around to my logic.* "The graduation won't last an hour. I'll be back before he misses me. He'll sleep the whole time."

Her eyes widen in disbelief. My heart falls. Little by little the reality drips into me, drop by drop like the liquids from my IV, and I slowly come to understand that I will miss Danny's kindergarten graduation. "He only graduates from kindergarten once in his whole life." My gaze stares straight ahead past the nurse. She says nothing.

It's not yet 8:00 in the morning and I've already cheated on my doctor, cost my husband and good friend a decent night's sleep, and now I'm neglecting Danny. How can one woman rack up so much failure before breakfast? Yet, the most precious bundle of newborn sweetness sleeps feet away. My oatmeal tastes like an odd mix of elation and defeat.

The nurse returns after breakfast and makes me lie on the bed, which is strange since I'm fully dressed including socks and shoes. She checks my pulse and presses her finger hard and deep into my abdomen. "Wow. Your uterus has gone down a lot. When did you deliver?"

"About 3:00 this morning." That's one thing in my favor. I have an incredible shrinking uterus. "What time does the pediatrician do his rounds? If the baby passes the tests, could we check out early?"

"They won't release you today," the nurse deadpans.

"Thought I'd ask."

She leaves, but I stay on the bed staring at the ceiling. At home I imagine Aaron is dashing around answering a volley of questions about the new baby and getting everyone dressed for graduation. They're all going without me. With nothing else to do, I project my mental budget onto the blank white ceiling, making neat columns of numbers. No epidural equals a savings of $500. Checking out in twenty-four rather than forty-eight hours will reduce the cost $1,000. Pain medicine won't be necessary—there's another couple hundred dollars. I scan the medical sales rack for any other deals.

After graduation, Aaron brings the kids to the hospital to meet their new brother. Danny is enthralled with baby Jack. He isn't upset in the least about me missing his graduation. This is bothering me a lot more than it's bothering him.

ON THURSDAY AFTERNOON, Aaron picks up Danny and Kate after their last half-day of school and brings them to the hospital to pick up Jack and me. A nurse enters my room pushing an empty wheelchair and looks around, taking in the odd spectacle of us. Aaron and I are standing in the center of the room loaded to the hilt like a couple of pack horses. Over his right elbow dangles tiny Jack buckled into the car seat. The space around Jack has been filled with newly acquired hospital accoutrements: free diaper bag, breast pump, formula samples, breastfeeding booklet, teddy bear, bulb syringe, and contraceptive information. With his left arm, Aaron balances two vases of flowers against his chest. Tanner is perched on my left hip; his tired head rests on my shoulder while he sucks his two middle fingers. He could care less about all this; he only wants his blankie and his crib. My right shoulder holds the weight of my overnight bag and purse. My hand is rendered unusable by Kate's death grip—she's overwhelmed by the sterile hospital environment, the machines and menacing contraptions. Danny is holding snug onto Kate's other hand.

The nurse folds down the footrests and pats the seat. "New mommy rides in a wheelchair. Hospital policy."

I give her a you've-got-to-be-kidding look that says something along the lines of *You may pretend to treat me like I'm all delicate and fragile by wheeling me out to the car, but sister, you and I both know that the second I get home I will walk myself into the house, start a load of laundry, answer the ringing phone, and defrost hamburger—all with this here infant attached to my chest—so let's put pretenses aside and let me just walk out of here.*

The nurse seems to consider the complex repacking and rearranging it will require for a five-minute ride. "Looks like you won't be needing this." She parks the wheelchair outside the door.

Signing my final release document requires prying Kate's fingers loose enough for me to hold the pen, then we all parade down the hallway dropping a trail of diaper rash samples behind us as we go.

At the entrance to Labor and Delivery, we pass Dr. Black, one of Dr. Woods' partners who I've seen for some of my prenatal visits. He looks at us quizzically, his eyes taking a moment to process the scene, then recognizes me as one of his patients.

"When did all this happen?" he asks in jest.

Mister, I wish you could tell me.

A FAMILY FROM church once confessed that their fourth child slept in a bottom dresser drawer for the first three months of his life until they could find one free hour on a Saturday to dig the crib out of the attic. At the time I vowed I would never be so unprepared. But—other than getting pregnant in the first place (and we're still a bit puzzled by that development, like a pair of guilty-looking thugs under questioning, "Honest officer, we don't know how it happened. We can't remember anything")—we haven't made any preparations for bringing Jack home. The outfit he's wearing, the baby blankets, burp cloths, car seat, and stroller, are passed down from Tanner. We do have a crib set up…if Tanner will move out of it.

The drive home from the hospital is deliciously peaceful. In the backseat Danny and Kate speak in sacred whispers as they watched their new brother yawn and twitch his little mouth. We should have stayed in the car. The moment we tote Jack through the front door, I answer three phone calls in a row and Aaron spends the afternoon responding to the doorbell. The Warner family merry-go-round is revolving at top speed and Jack has been pulled into the spin. The reason babies projectile vomit on every article of clothing a mother owns has nothing to do with milk or acid reflux, it's the sheer nature of the speed of life.

And speaking of milk, mine hasn't come in yet, but I set up breastfeeding basecamp on our family room sectional. The pull-down console pocket gets stocked with nursing pads, burp rags, diapers, wipes, and back issues of *Reader's Digest*. Once Danny and Kate finish lunch, they spread a blanket on the family room floor with Jack in the middle surrounded by stuffed animals and toys. While Tanner naps, Jack becomes the center of their play.

Sometime during all this I get a message that Laiah is coming to Phoenix for a work assignment, the length of which has yet to be determined. She's exploring housing options. With the new baby she wants to be close and spend as much time with me as possible. I let her know she is welcome to stay anytime and remind her that we'll be spending most of the summer in Utah. "I have a lot of work in Utah this summer as well," she informs me.

FRIDAY MORNING, AARON and I open our eyes to see a crowd of baby brother fans lined up next to our bed before sunrise in hopes of getting a glimpse of the new family celebrity. They've already checked the carrier and found it empty. Jack is sleeping next to me. No reason to move Tanner out of the crib when we'll be leaving home in a few weeks anyway. "Hop up here." I pat the bed.

Danny and Kate jump up and snuggle in. Kate rubs Jack's head. Danny coaxes Jack's hand to open and grip his finger. "He sure is press-us." Kate kisses Jack's head over and over. "Hi Jack. It's me. It's your sister Katie." Her smile fills the room. "He's just a little bit cute. Sure is." She examines his tiny toes.

"Kate, will you watch Jack carefully while I go to the bathroom?" My body protests against the act of standing up. Sitting on the toilet I dread releasing the stream of morning urine which burns the stretched, ripped, raw skin. There must be a lot of stitches, but I don't want to know what it looks like down there. In the shower I carefully wash around the IV bruise, scrubbing away the sticky tape residue. Under the warm water, my breasts tingle and swell—my milk is coming in faster than I expected. The tingle isn't painful, but it doesn't feel good.

By noon my milk is flowing with a vengeance. Bringing Jack close to nurse is like holding his face to a spraying fire hydrant. If only nipples came with dials to control the flow. Jack can't eat a fraction of the supply available to him. When he's swallowed more than his fill, I wonder if there are any starving puppies in the neighborhood—I could sustain a litter or two as well as a fleet of Meadow Gold ice cream trucks.

Friday afternoon, Annice picks up Mom and our baby sister Deedee from the airport. Aaron carries my mom's luggage into the house. She has two suitcases: one for her personal items and another full of quilting and crocheting projects to keep her busy while she's here. Mom, Annice, Deedee, and I chat while the cousins play in the backyard. We talk and my mom's hands are always busy. She is crocheting a light blue baby afghan for Jack. Kate brings Deedee flowers picked from our hibiscus plants. Deedee rises to her status as favorite aunt. The kids adore her attention.

"Why don't you go rest and we'll watch the kids," Annice tells me.

But this is rare time to be with my mom and sisters with no pesky brothers dominating the conversation with sports and politics, or my dad rehashing old stories. Today I have these favorite women all to myself. "I'm not tired. I don't want to miss out on the conversation."

Over the next few hours, Jack eats so little and my breasts continue to swell. I made the mistake of wearing an underwire bra because it was the only one that would fit, and by Saturday I'm spiking a fever. Double mastitis. Hard, red nodules lump under the skin. Jack can't drain the excess. The only solution is to hook up an electric pump in order to suck open the clogged ducts, allowing fresh milk to flow through and wash out the infection. In the pharmacy the handheld pump looked so innocuous. Now it's a yellow torture device approaching my tender nipples like a hooded executioner. Tears pour down my face. I can hardly force myself to do the other side. When both bottles are completely full, I walk to my bathroom sink and pour the creamy contents down the drain, watching it spiral in a milky swirl like the top of a soft ice cream cone. My body works round the clock concocting that particular recipe with special DHA and antibodies. The white liquid disappears down the pipe where it will mix with the dirty dishwater and someone's diarrhea. Shaking the bottles empty, I cry over spilled milk.

CHAPTER 18

The Retreat

IN 1917, THE Goodyear Tire and Rubber Company purchased sixteen thousand acres of land in south-central Arizona. The company had made two discoveries. One, that adding cotton extended the life and wear of tires. Two, that central Arizona—with its Egypt-like climate—was an excellent place to grow cotton. Thus, the city of Goodyear, Arizona was born. After six months selling ads to nearly every business in the Goodyear area, I'm getting familiar with its layout and history. The tire company built guest houses to host visiting executives and those guest houses grew into what became a five-star resort called the Wigwam. This summer, Aaron's company is hosting the annual Cloverman family retreat at the Wigwam Resort.

Jack is two weeks and one day old, buckled into his car seat with the shade visor pulled over to protect his delicate, new skin. His chin droops on his chest, his knees tuck up to his belly. He still defaults to fetal position, making him look like a head of cabbage. He's parked next to the back tire while I stuff luggage under the minivan's raised back door: swimsuits, sunscreen, life preservers, inflatable inner tubes, water sandals, sunhats, snacks, dinner outfits, plus the endless catalogue of baby paraphernalia. We're only going for three days and we're packed floor to roof. After driving thirty minutes, Aaron unlocks the door to our cottage. Kate, Danny, and Tanner race into the room, find their swimsuits, and beg to go swimming. The company family retreat has begun.

Aaron leaves for his opening meetings. I chase the kids to the pool awkwardly holding Jack's carrier to my chest, the heavy shoulder bag bouncing as I run. Mostly I'm praying to be able to keep track of all four of them by the water.

Positioning Jack under an umbrella and arranging our towels on pool chairs has me worked into a sweat. My breast milk virtually evaporates into the arid June sky. Just then Laiah sneaks up behind me. She's arranged her schedule to spend the afternoon at the pool with us.

"Get a gander at all the peacocks strutting their newest developments." Laiah draws my attention to the other Cloverman wives setting up around the pool. This year I have a rack to rival the most surgically enhanced, but considering the general sag, jiggle, and pasty whiteness of everything from my neck down, the only sashaying I do will be between this chair and the restroom to change my pads. Otherwise, I plan to sit in this corner wearing my black swim cover-up.

"Check out Veronica." Laiah lets out a low whistle. Across the way Veronica is setting up a shade tent looking flawless. She is beautifully tan and wearing (of all things!) a white bikini the exact color of my skin. "Doesn't she have four kids same as you? You can't tell by looking at her. Remember last year when we visited her new house?"

Of course I remember. Veronica had opened the door wearing an apron over an outfit that could have come straight off a New York runway. She was in the middle of baking homemade pies. She amicably stopped her work and escorted us through a tour, showing the window treatments she had sewn herself. "I found the fabric on clearance. It saved us thousands of dollars." Pulling out a measuring stick and comparing the two of us, I came out much shorter.

My inferiority complex is interrupted by Kate's yell from across the pool. Tanner has flipped face forward in his swim tube and is splashing and gurgling, unable to right himself. Without thinking about not getting my stitches wet, I jump into the water, run-swim across the pool and lift Tanner's face out of the water. He coughs and starts to cry. My heart thumps in my ears. How did I allow myself to get distracted and nearly lose my son? I pull him close to my chest and rub his head, then lift him to the side of the pool to dry him off. As I heft myself up out of the water, my episiotomy pops. Skin opens. All the commotion wakes Jack, whose cries cause my milk to let down. Thankfully I'm already wet, so the circles of milk aren't too noticeable through my swimsuit.

All the immaculate women are watching us. Kate is crying. Tanner is crying. Jack is crying. I am springing leaks and trying not to cry. The threads holding me together are coming unstitched. I am falling apart at the seams.

—⟞⟝—

AS THE RETREAT progresses, the lines at the buffets grow shorter. At each meal we make note of who's missing. Whispers through the food lines speculate about hotel food poisoning or an uber-contagious stomach flu. By the third day of the company retreat, anyone who hasn't already vomited is cautiously waiting to see who it strikes next. We make it to Saturday unscathed. While Aaron delivers our three amigos to kids' camp, I dress for the final awards banquet. No one here with Cloverman knows yet, but this is our last summer retreat and awards banquet. Come Monday, Aaron will officially resign as a financial advisor to come home and join me full-time on our printing business. This year we aren't worried about making impressions, which is good because the only formal attire my mega-boobs fit into is an old sweater with a few sparkling sequins. Aaron returns to our room and tells me I look beautiful.

At dinner, Aaron and I clink glasses with our table companions and toast to a great year at Cloverman. Under the table we take turns rocking Jack's carrier with our toes to keep him sleeping. Twelve months have ticked past since last year's banquet. We have a business and a baby—both were so unpredictable and already so obviously normal it's hard to imagine that neither existed a brief year ago. How can life be so extraordinary and mundane at once?

After the award presentations, Aaron and I pick up our troops from kids' camp. Wired on sugar and lack of sleep, they jump from one hotel bed to the other.

"Should we pack up and go home to our own beds?" Aaron asks, surveying the scene.

"It will take longer to get them settled down to sleep than it will for us to drive back home. If somebody starts puking tonight, I'd rather be home with my own washing machine."

MONDAY MORNING AARON kisses me goodbye and leaves to clean out his office and tie up any loose ends for his last day of work. Meanwhile in the laundry room, four heaping piles of laundry wait to be washed, dried, folded, and repacked into the same suitcases so we can leave for Utah tomorrow. I strip our bed sheets and add them to the rest of the wash. Laiah's always had this thing about never leaving home with dirty sheets on the beds and it's spread to me. "What if the house caught fire and the firefighters rushed in and could smell stale sheets over the stench of smoke?" Tomorrow I'll wash the kids' sheets before we leave.

In the pre-dawn hours early Tuesday morning, Danny mopes into our bedroom. "Mom, I don't feel good." His face is pale with a hint of green. He hiccups. The moment I see his stomach muscles contract, I dive-roll into Aaron as Danny heaves forward, depositing a pile of brown puke exactly where I'd been lying.

"That's slow-reacting food poisoning." Aaron looks over me at the stinking mass. "That or it's stomach flu."

"I think they're allergic to the laundry detergent." I scoot closer to Aaron.

"Why?"

"Because they only throw up on freshly washed sheets." The sheets on Danny's own bed are dirty, but he had made it all the way into our bedroom to throw up all over the only clean sheets in the house. We both roll out of Aaron's side of the bed. Aaron fetches the barf bowl for Danny and tucks him back to bed while I strip our sheets for the second day in a row.

Tanner vomits next, followed by Kate and we postpone our departure a couple of days. Instead of arriving in Utah with time to get settled and recuperate from our ten-hour drive, we will pull into town the night before Aaron's brother's wedding and hope we don't spread flu germs to the bride and groom.

CHAPTER 19

Why?

LATE FRIDAY NIGHT, I'm awake rocking a fussy Jack in the downstairs of Aaron's childhood home. Between the dark hours of midnight and pre-dawn, my bare feet wear the pattern of waltz steps into the old, shag carpet. Poor Jack. He's overstimulated after being passed to so many unfamiliar arms during the wedding celebrations. The combination of his empty stomach and strange surroundings result in an inconsolable baby who cries the moment I try to lay him down. We become acquainted with midnight shadows cast through the basement window.

The wedding day ended with a spectacular demonstration from Tanner, who had discovered that reception ennui could be averted by throwing Rice Krispy balls into the chocolate fountain in the same way a boring day of fishing is fixed by throwing rocks into the water. His flailing arms spewed splatters of chocolate onto the white linens as I pulled him away from the refreshment table igniting a no-afternoon-nap-meltdown-tantrum, showcasing a spectacle of body-writhing, kicking, screaming, and hair-pulling (mine *and* his) to rival the most brutal exorcism. Somehow the bride escaped without brown chocolate spots on her white gown.

A nauseous stomach also keeps me awake—hard to know whether it's the Cloverman retreat stomach flu or a ten-hour drive followed by too much wedding dessert and birthday cake—but several times the gut rumbling sends me running to the bathroom where I must set Jack on the cold linoleum in order to lean over the porcelain bowl. Thus I pass the night pacing the hallway, bouncing Jack against my chest, and cradling his head into my shoulder to soothe and also muffle the volume so his crying wouldn't wake my in-laws.

Thankfully I never throw up—this is the good news. Nobody wants to finish their birthday by vomiting into a toilet. I turned thirty-one years today. Somehow, Aaron managed to stop by a grocery store and bring a surprise, store-bought birthday cake to the wedding luncheon, which—if you think about it—was a waste of money since there was already dessert provided by the caterers. In the midst of a bustling day, Helen also remembered my birthday and gave me a card.

Sometime later, I hear the ruckus of the Danny-Kate-Tanner trio upstairs. At last I've fallen asleep on the family room couch, Jack sleeping curled on my chest. The adults in the house want to sleep late after a long day of wedding festivities, but my kids bounce awake at 6:30 a.m. no matter how late they went to bed. They sound like a herd of elephants running through the kitchen, dumping out Grandma's toys, and raiding her cereal closet. I should bring them downstairs so they don't wake Helen and Grant, but...Jack is *sleeping*. My eyes close and I drift back to sleep listening to the sound of Helen's voice asking the trio what they want for breakfast.

It's late when I slide Jack onto the couch and go to the bathroom to splash cold water over my eyes, blink out the redness, and carry Jack upstairs. Before entering the living room, I tilt my chin up and put on a smile. "Good morning everybody."

Helen moves out of her recliner. "Sit down here." She pats the cushion for me then takes a seat on the floor.

"We are going to hike up Payson Canyon. How long until you can be ready?" Aaron's words highlight the fact that I'm the only person in the room still wearing pajamas.

Hiking? I could barely walk up the stairs.

"Go ahead. I'll stay here." Under the blanket I lift my shirt and help Jack latch on.

Aaron looks crushed. "Why?"

Why?!

The room waits for me to answer, but my brain struggles to formulate a coherent response. Saying "I'm tired" is no good—everybody is tired after yesterday. I wish I could be more organized and on top of everything as other women are. I wish I could bound out of bed ready to spend the day on a grand hiking adventure. But today is Saturday, and there's something pressing I need to do. Through my grogginess, I can't come up with it. My brain is swimming in letters, like alphabet soup, but I can't turn the stew into words. In the end, the only word I find is a word that means everything and nothing.

"Because."

The word doesn't satisfy.

"I'll carry Jack for you." Aaron knows he has a solution to fix this problem.

"He was so fussy last night. I think he needs to stay in one place today."

"I'll stay home and watch him while you go." Now Helen has the fix.

"Please come. Please come," Danny and Kate sing in chorus.

In the pause I'm taken back to the hospital the day Jack was born—the yearning to be at Danny's graduation, the desire to divide myself into more than one person. Everyone is looking at me.

"I can't."

"Why?" Aaron questions again.

"Don't you want to go?" Grant asks. "I'll help with the kids."

There is nothing to do but shake my head. They pack water, snacks, and sunscreen and ask three more times if I'm sure, before leaving me sitting in the front room questioning if I made the right decision. Rather than going back downstairs to rest while the house is quiet, I sit on the couch, awkwardly glancing at *why?*

I hate that Aaron invited *why?* here this morning—a demanding houseguest—and left me alone to entertain him.

Why? hovers in the room looking at family photos on the mantle, drawing fingerprints in the dust on the fireplace, scrutinizing me over his double monocles. He pinches both pant legs, hiking the trousers above sock level before lowering himself onto the far end of the couch. "Hmph," he torts while polishing his lenses.

I tell myself to ignore *why?*, but he is so curious, so interesting. There's much he could reveal to me: *Why* wasn't I able to go hiking with my family? *Why* aren't I capable of doing everything that everyone thinks I should be able to do? *Why* am I weaker than other women?

I examine *why?* for clues while thinking about all the days backward: the hike, the wedding, the ten-hour drive, the puke-soiled bed sheets, the company family retreat, my mom and sister's visit, Jack's birth...

Why doesn't Aaron realize it's all been too much? *Why* wouldn't he tell me to stay home and rest? *Why* doesn't he see how exhausted I am? *Why* did my in-laws think I should be able to go hiking the day after a big wedding, which was the day after a long car drive, which was barely three weeks after giving birth to their grandson?

And before that was the music conference, the long drive to Tucson... Before that was the June magazine deadline, the months of door-to-door selling, piano lessons, seminary, cleaning out the family house... I think all the way back to that night when Aaron left me sitting alone at the awards banquet.

"*Why* is it never enough?" I shout out loud.

I want to cry—a deep, cleansing cry while the house is mine alone. I want to sob hard, washing away the *why?* until I am purged. But tears don't come on demand. *Why?* presses his hands to his knees, raises himself with importance, and exits the front door without asking to be excused. What poor manners! He robbed the peaceful hours of my morning and gave nothing in return. He may answer to his name, but he doesn't have answers to his name.

I'm left alone sitting on the couch; Jack has long since fallen back to sleep. In the quiet, the nagging feeling of an unremembered task resurfaces. *What is it I needed to do today?*

A sound outside calls my attention. "Knock, knock? Hello?" Laiah breezes in. She is in town for something important, but at this moment I can't recall what exactly. "I can only stay a minute." She takes *why?*'s place on the couch and looks around, noticing the quiet. "Where is everybody?"

"They went hiking. Please don't ask me *why* I didn't go. Just tell me *why* I'm not as strong as people think I should be. Helen fed my kids breakfast this morning. I'm a horrible mother."

It's barely 9:00 on a Saturday morning and Laiah is dressed for business, giving the impression she's already completed a number of significant accomplishments for the day. After Kate was born, I'd asked her if there were mothering judges or a mothering report card. How else does a woman know if she's succeeding in mothering? I need a way to know if I'm doing things right. Laiah could be my guide. She works as a consultant or a coach (I don't understand her work exactly). She's successful, organized, put-together, a dynamo—all the things I'm not. Now that she's living close by, would she do it? Will she help me organize my life? Will she show me where I'm falling short and tell me how to fix it? Will she help me be successful?

"Yes." Laiah nods. "I'll do whatever you want. I'm here for you."

I've seen the personal evaluation forms she carries around where people can self-assess their competence in areas like timeliness, organization, reliability, and preparedness. I need her to point out where I'm falling short and tell me how to fix it. I need her to coach me on how to be successful.

"First, tell me where I went wrong this morning. How did I let so many people down?"

"Did you sleep late?" Laiah and I have had a thing since college about not wasting life by sleeping in: *Early to bed, early to rise. The little bird who wakes up early is healthy, wealthy and gets the fattest worm.*

"Yes. I slept late. I heard the kids awake then I let myself fall back to sleep."

"Helen had a wedding yesterday and is probably even more exhausted than you are. Here's the thing. Life is hard. Everybody gets tired. You have to be stronger than your body and force yourself to get up and get moving."

Laiah is right. If I'd gotten up the first time I'd heard the kids wake, I could have fed them breakfast—like a good mother would do—and been dressed and ready to go on the hike.

"No person ever achieved success by keeping company with their pillow."

Did Laiah hear that from a philosopher, a self-help guru, or did she make it up?

The back screen door slams, letting in a cacophony of voices and announcing the triumphal return of the hiking expedition. The conquering heroes regale tales of snake catching and wading under the waterfall. Their sun-kissed faces are luminous with the excitement of adventure. They crawl their gangly bodies onto my lap, wrap their rangy appendages around my neck and show me pictures from Aaron's camera of mountain cows and meadow flowers. I can feel their heartbeats pulsing warm and alive in their necks.

"You are cold!" Kate tells me and retracts from my embrace. She asks why I'm still wearing pajamas, why I'm sitting in the same place I was when they left. Kate plays with my hand while she talks about racing sticks down the river and asks why the veins on my wrist are blue and flat. She doesn't expect me to answer, which I don't, not out loud. *My veins are empty*, I think. *No lifeblood there*. My morning has been an utter waste—first, sleeping late, then squandering precious time bickering with *why?* Their outing had been fantastic and while they have memories and sunburns, I have regret. Three hours of hiking would have been a cinch compared to my morning wrestling with guilt. I should have gone. I made the wrong decision. For the rest of the summer, I vow to myself, I will participate in anything and everything my family wants to do.

Helen interrupts my thoughts. "What can I do to help for tomorrow?"

What's tomorrow? Seconds tick off in my brain to the backdrop of quiz show music before the answer to my nagging feeling finally surfaces.

Tomorrow is Sunday. Jack's blessing day.

CHAPTER 20

Blessing Day

TOMORROW THERE WILL be forty-plus extended family and friends gathered at a special church service to witness Jack's baby blessing, which is like a Catholic christening but without the godparents or the baptism. Afterward this crowd of forty will be *hungry*, and whose job will it be to feed them?

Mine.

I wonder if other postpartum Mormon mothers around the world, like me, are planning food, rounding up extra tables and chairs, and prepping to feed a Mormon army. Tanner's blessing was held in Arizona and Annice volunteered to host the luncheon at her house and to cook all the food. (I enjoyed the day immensely.) But since we're already in Utah for the wedding, and most of our family is here (everyone except Annice, ironically) we decided to have Jack's blessing at my parents' church in Salt Lake City. This infelicitous conglomeration of events requires me to organize a transportable celebration. Even at home with my own pots and pans I'm a shaky meal planner. Hosting has never been my strong suit. Working with borrowed kitchen utensils pilfered from Helen's cupboards, I need to prepare a meal that can be hauled to the reception room of my parent's condo building. The food must stay warm—or cold, as needed—during the service and be ready to serve the minute church ends. Also, the cost must remain below budget.

"What can I do to help?" Helen asks again.

"I think I've got it covered." (Translation: I have *nothing* planned.) "Could I borrow your slow cooker?"

That afternoon Aaron pulls van keys from his pocket so I can go to Costco. I'd cornered him alone downstairs. "We need to decide what we're serving for lunch tomorrow," I fire at him.

This was news to him, up to that point he'd been unaware such a decision existed. "Isn't everybody bringing something?"

"Yes, everyone is bringing potluck salads and desserts, but we need to provide the main dish…and drinks!"

"Let's get meat and cheese trays." Aaron has the resolution to the dilemma.

"That would be the easiest, but it would be expensive. Shredded pork would be less expensive and it would be more formal."

"Do pork then," Aaron answers simply.

But it isn't simple. Grabbing Laiah to come along, we drive to the Provo Costco, and on the way try to remember the recipe to Annice's special Sunday pork roast, then graph how many pounds of meat will fit in a standard crock pot. "Is it one-quarter pound of meat serving per person? That doesn't sound like enough. Maybe it's one-half pound per person? No, that sounds like too much." While I attempt to calculate, Laiah makes a list of my sisters-in-law who live the closest so I can call to borrow their slow cookers.

We traipse to the back of Costco and scour the meat chests, but the Provo store doesn't carry the same pork product as my Glendale store. Can I buy the pork at a grocery store? Laiah asks. But I don't know what *kind* of pork I get from Costco: pork loin roast, pork butt roast, pork shoulder roast, pork shoulder butt, pork belly, pork rinds… All I know is my cart swings past the meat section, my hand grabs the pork—packaged three per pack—from the end chest, because that's where Annice told me to find it, then I push my cart into the dairy freezer to grab milk. Butchers go to school to learn the various cuts of meat. The only thing I know about meat is that other women's pork roasts turn out tender, juicy, and delicious and mine are dry, chewy, and tasteless, *unless* I use this particular pork from Costco. Substituting grocery store pork is too risky.

Laiah and I drive along back roads hammering out the pros and cons of other edible options. "You've had nine months to prepare for this blessing and you're just now getting around to planning food?"

"I know. I know." It's not that I haven't thought about it. I've lost sleep fretting about this meal, but like most things, the fretting didn't lead to getting anything done. Laiah doesn't even have to say how I'd score on *preparedness*. Jack's baby blessing is like the ultimate test of all the mothering skills I'm supposed to possess: planning, decorating, cooking, hosting, taking care of everyone's needs, and doing it all with poise, grace, a smile on my face, and a body that "doesn't look like you had a baby three weeks ago." Everyone will be watching to see how I manage the day, and by everyone, I mean all the mothering judges. I thought the judges would ease off once I started working the magazine and became more than just a stay-at-home mom, but on the contrary, the pressure is higher to see how I'm managing adding a fourth baby and running a business. The meal should be somewhat fancy. I can't throw out hot dogs and bags of potato chips on a plastic table cover. What would people think?

Delicious food, transferable pots, cheap and elegant—the conditions are too complicated under the best of circumstances and here I am with boobs hard as coconuts, my cha-chi stitched in the pattern of a French landmark, and my hormones teetering between depletion and surging. With hands trembling around the steering wheel, I turn by mistake onto a long, unpaved road that takes me east toward the mountains, a long way from where I need to be. My heart beats in my throat. My mental circuits are shorting out. I am sizzling, sparking, threatening to explode.

Hours later, Laiah and I return emptyhanded.

It's late when Aaron walks me to the deli counter of the local grocery store where I stare blankly—like a wounded vet with posttraumatic stress disorder—at the varieties of meats. The meats and cheeses are on sale. In the end, Aaron places the order for a tally less than the cost of pork roast. Fifteen minutes and the task is done. Too easily we slide the prepared trays in the fridge and go to bed, when I expected to be awake all night seasoning, cooking, and shredding pork.

THE DAY AFTER Jack's blessing, the kids want to meet up with cousins at a dinosaur park. I want one day to recuperate, but remembering the hike I say, "Sure."

For the rest of the summer we visit museums and waterparks and go see the wild buffalo on Antelope Island. We go to outdoor concerts and indoor playgrounds. We end July by doing the perfect activity for a woman sporting more pads than the Kotex aisle at Walmart. We go camping.

At my Big Mormon Family Reunion, Kate finds me seated on a couch in a corner of the lodge and lays her head on the part of my lap not occupied by Jack. I extend his blanket to cover her shoulders. "Are you worn out from all the commotion, little bitty?" She nods and I smooth her hair and caress her cheeks. In no time she is sound asleep, snoring loudly.

My cousin, Trinity, walks toward me. "Is this the napping couch? I could use a nap." Trinity moves a pillow and sits. "Is Kate making that noise?"

"She always snores like this," I say.

"I thought it was the air conditioner." Trinity leans over Kate and studies her breathing. "Does she have big tonsils?"

"Huge," I answer. "Her tonsils cover the back of her throat. I don't know how she can swallow anything."

"She sounds like my oldest. Anna used to snore so loud we had to wear earplugs at night."

"What did you do?"

"Ear, nose, and throat specialist. Took out her tonsils, adenoids, and put in ear tubes. Best thing we ever did. She sleeps so quiet now, I check to make sure she's breathing. No more purple bags under her eyes and more energy for school."

Kate's ragged breathing and purple eye rings have worried me for a while, but I've asked every pediatrician and they insist she's fine. Trinity's comments reaffirm that Kate is not fine and when we get back to Arizona, I will be looking for a good ear, nose and throat specialist.

CHAPTER 21

Burning Up On Reentry

THE SKYLINE ABOVE the Rocky Mountains is dark and speckled with morning stars as Aaron pulls the van onto the road. Somewhere in that vast sky, the International Space Station hovers, the astronauts sip morning coffee through a straw inserted into an airtight plastic bag, gazing at earth and watching one of the sixteen sunrises or sunsets that marks one day in space. They gaze at earth as I gaze at the stars. Twelve years earlier, the Honorable Senator Jake Garn spoke to my college about his voyage as the first member of congress to space. He said the beauty of the earth from space is impossible to describe, but he must have described it in exquisite detail because I sat in the lecture hall enraptured by a vision of earth all green and blue with a halo-like glow, as if the planet herself were a celestial being with aura, intelligence, and spirit. An angel. Mother Earth. No political boundaries, no war zones, no prisons, only the glory and perfection of earth's pure potential without the clutter of human failings. This is how I feel leaning my forehead against the cool, dew-misted passenger window, listening to the low hum of the van engine. I am orbiting my life, hovering in the space between our summer moon and our return to planet earth, hoping we don't burn up on reentry.

Aaron steers the van through the streets of downtown Salt Lake City, then accelerates, climbing the on-ramp for southbound I-15. Only 421 miles to Las Vegas. Tilting my head against the cool window, I watch my breath form clouds on the glass. I will miss the cool, crisp Utah mornings. The only thing crisp about Arizona summer mornings is the bacon you can fry on the hood of your car for breakfast. In the back seat, Kate and Danny lean together, supporting each other's weight with a pillow in between. Tanner has fallen asleep sucking his two middle fingers, his head leaned against the side of his car seat. Jack sucks his thumb. There's no telling how long this rare delicacy of silence will last.

This summer has been everything we've wanted for our kids: adventure, outdoor exploration, night games, and no backyard fences. Now we need routine. Jack needs his own bed. We all do. Most of all I look forward to nursing Jack in the open privacy of my own home without worrying about a brother-in-law catching a glimpse of exposed breast. We have experienced a child's dream summer; now it's time for Aaron and me to start living our dream.

A smile turns up my lips as I realize that starting Monday morning, Aaron will no longer go to an office, leaving me home feeling isolated and trapped within my own four walls until 5:00 p.m. He will be home to help with the morning routine—breakfast, finding shoes, brushing teeth, scrubbing spilled toothpaste out of carpet. I won't have to find a babysitter for dentist appointments or when I volunteer in Danny's classroom. He'll be home in the afternoon so I can teach a full, uninterrupted thirty-minute piano lesson while Aaron refills sippy cups, changes stinky diapers, and—a jolt of giddiness leaps from my chest—*makes dinner*. Aaron and I have talked about working together from home for years and now it's finally happening. My smile grows full-sized and spreads up my cheeks, changing the shape of the exhalation clouds on the window.

"What's wrong?" Aaron asks about the strange sound escaping my throat.

I reach over and touch his leg softly. "Nothing. I'm thinking about Monday when you, Mr. Warner, do *not* have to go to work." I pat his knee silently, but with the vigor of a congratulatory handshake. "What do you think about that?"

"It's weird. I'm excited." His eyes sparkle and my smile spreads to his lips.

We share smiles, each tickled with our own little fantasies of what Monday means. I'm thinking how Aaron will teach me layout and design, which I will do from our home office in between feeding Jack while he takes over the pavement-pounding ad sales job. I'll venture down to Goodyear once, maybe twice a week, to meet with my current customers and maybe sell a new ad here and there, but I'm happy to let Aaron take over worrying about increasing our advertising revenue. He is the trained salesman.

In my mind, Aaron is envisioning the exact dream that I am, but when he speaks, he talks about something else entirely. "Did I tell you about my new business idea?" he whispers.

"Which one?" I tease. If he had a dozen Methuselah lifetimes, Aaron couldn't touch a fraction of his business brainstorms. Monday is a sort of Independence Day for Aaron. He will have eight hours of unscheduled, unobligated daytime hours to pursue ideas that have been simmering on his brain's back burner for the past six years. His eyes practically shine with the prospects of his newfound freedom.

This long drive would be the perfect opportunity for Aaron and me to plan our new life. With hours to talk, we could set boundaries, clarify expectations, divide household chores, and designate office hours. Who will get Danny and Kate ready for school, do Tanner's morning routine, drive carpool, fix meals, wash dishes, oversee naptime, help with homework, be on-call for emergencies? I'm ready for life to settle down. Starting Monday, Aaron will be home to help manage the herd and I can step back from the harrowing pace of the past six months. But it never occurs to either of us to have that conversation. We are both riding confidently on the presumption that, come Monday, we are finally going to have exactly what we've each wanted.

So when Danny and Kate wake up and beg for the audiobook, we oblige. This summer we've passed the miles across Utah and Idaho by listening to Lemony Snicket's *A Series of Unfortunate Events*. It's a colorfully deplorable children's tale about the Baudelaire orphans who are left in the care of a sequence of bumbling adults who should be all the wiser about the obvious trouble before their eyes, but who—for various reasons—remain ignorant to the children's cues for help. We left off with the Baudelaire orphans watching their Aunt Josephine disappear into the dark, leech-infested waters of Lake Lachrymose with Count Olaf and silly Mr. Poe waiting to ship them off to their next distant relative. Aaron presses the play button, adjusts the volume; all is silent. From the back I can practically hear Kate and Danny holding their breath, wondering why the CD isn't playing yet. The seconds pass and the tires churn the road beneath us as we wait for the narrator to reveal the next series of unfortunate events.

CHAPTER 22

The Longest Day (reprise)

MONDAY MORNING LAIAH rides in the car with me when I drive Danny and Kate to their first day of school. She'd come over the night before and we'd talked so late that she ended up staying.

Danny jumps out of the car and runs to his classroom before I can hug him. "Have a great day in first grade!" I shout, waving until he disappears inside the door. I hold Kate's hand and walk her to the kindergarten building. She wriggles free of my grip and runs ahead.

"Bye Mom." Kate skips through the kindergarten door without looking back. Outside I press my hands against the window, peering inside the classroom to see if she seems nervous. What if she doesn't know what to do? Other parents join me until a teacher's aide comes to the door and asks us to leave because we are distracting the students. Laiah laughs, razzing me about being one of those sappy mothers who boo-hoos when her baby starts school.

Opening my front door reveals an entirely different kitchen from the one I left. The contents of the toy cupboard are spread across the living room, kitchen, and family room. Tanner is awake. He has taken off his pajamas and sits top and center of the kitchen table. His overnight diaper leaves wet streaks as he scoots and spins up and down the table, spilling soggy cereal from his loosely-held bowl. From the bedroom comes the sound of Jack's hungry morning cry.

"Jack is crying," I call to Aaron while washing sticky milk off Tanner's hands, face, and bare tummy. My dream of having Aaron home in the morning to help get the kids ready for school hadn't panned out today. When his alarm rang, he'd headed straight for the shower, gotten dressed, and shut himself in the office. What he's working on in there is a mystery. Maybe it's habit, waking up and going to an office.

Tanner is tucked under my arm like a sack of flour, kicking and protesting against getting dressed. He's mastered taking off his pajamas at night and he fights wearing clothing during the day. It's August in Arizona—who can blame him?

"Can you hear Jack crying?" I peek my head into the office to see Aaron working on the computer. His eyes never leave the screen.

"I heard you," Aaron calls back. "There's nothing I can do for him when he's hungry."

"Maybe you could change diapers?" I grumble to myself.

In the bedroom, my knee pins Tanner to the floor while I wrestle to change his diaper. He is not trapped in a car seat today and all he wants to do is *run*. Once he's dressed I set him free to play. Jack's diaper is also soggy, the excess urine leaving an oval puddle on my side of the bed. The wet diaper is a good sign he's getting enough to eat. Traveling always dries my milk. We've been home two days and my supply is getting stronger.

Laiah watches me give Jack a bath. I fill a washcloth with water and let the drops trickle a path up his poochy baby tummy and chest until the drips tease the corners of Jack's mouth. He flicks out his little tongue. A miss-aimed drop lands square in his eyes. He winces, blinks, and sneezes.

"What are you going to do today?" Laiah asks.

If it were up to me, I would freeze this moment scooping warm water over Jack's chunky legs, but Bob is coming for a business meeting and piano lessons resume this afternoon. "I need to ask Aaron to clean up the kitchen before Bob gets here." I hold tight to Jack's slippery body with one arm while enwrapping him in a towel with the other.

"Wait," Laiah stops me. "It's Aaron's kitchen as much as yours. It's not *your* job to ask him to help *you* clean *his* kitchen. You're both working the magazine now. He should know he needs to do household chores." We carry Jack's clothes and baby lotion past the office door, saying nothing, and settle on the family room couch to get Jack dressed and give him his morning feeding.

I've just switched Jack to the other breast when Aaron's quick footsteps click across the tile. In one continual motion he scans the disastrous state of the kitchen, from the cereal-filled milk puddle on the table to the half-wall where Tanner is launching matchbox cars. His eyes land on me. I'm wearing cut-off sweats with my feet propped up on the footrest, singing a leisurely song to Jack.

"Bob is going to be here in twenty minutes!" Aaron leaps into missile mode clearing the table, loading the dishwasher, sweeping the floor. He polishes the table, scrubs dried milk drips off the chairs and digs a tablecloth from the back of a cupboard. Tanner is banished to the garage-turned-playroom, chastised for making the mess. Aaron throws toys into the cupboard, every now and then shooting a glance my way.

"Wow. Did you see the glare Aaron launched this way?" Laiah points out. "You could slice glaciers with that torpedo."

I've been awake for three hours and have fed and dressed four humans, but this is the first time Aaron has seen me today. Why am I the one feeling guilty—while sitting on the couch nursing *our* eight-week-old son—that Aaron is helping with *my* work and not vice versa?

"You'll have to finish later, little man." My finger in the corner of his mouth breaks the suction. I dash down the hall cradling Jack, who looks confused by the abrupt end to his meal. Placing him in the middle of my bed, I scour the closet to find some non-maternity business attire to wear. The doorbell rings. Aaron greets Bob and invites him in. Running down the hall, my fingers swoop my hair into a hasty ponytail.

Bob takes my extended hand and pulls me and Jack to his chest. He's the same age as my dad and his warm hug engulfs me. "Welcome back. How's the baby doing?" Bob examines Jack. "He has grown over the summer."

He *has* grown. The first two months of Jack's life are gone. The thought wrings my heart.

At the kitchen table, Bob lays out copies of our April, May, and June issues. Aaron's cover designs look sharp lined up in a row. For April and May he chose stock images, but the June cover is Aaron's own nature photography. This magazine and Jack are the same age. I was pregnant with both at once, but rather than relishing a sense of accomplishment, I'm holding my breath waiting to hear Bob's prospectus regarding our startup months. He has the numbers. He knows if we ended profitable or in the hole. At last he sets both hands on the table. "Well…I think the first three issues turned out fine." He reaches into his accordion folder and hands us copies of June's review sheet with the breakdown of advertising income and business expenses. "We didn't make money, but we didn't lose money either."

Out of the thirty-two advertisers, sixteen were new accounts I had landed, including the highest paying ad. I hadn't known if I would be able to do it, but I had sold enough advertising to cover the printing and mailing expenses for all three issues. Not bad for a pregnant lady cold-contacting business owners during preschool hours. Those five months had been grueling. I wait for Aaron or Bob to mention the amazing work I'd done getting the magazine off the ground. Bob looks my way and I'm ready for his verbal pat on the back. Instead he asks, "How many of your existing customers are planning to advertise in the September issue?"

"Um, I haven't contacted any of them yet." I fumble for the right words. "We got back Saturday and I had to get the kids ready to start school…"

Jack sneezes loudly and we all turn to look. The noise disrupted his sleep and he cries to be consoled. Bob pauses the meeting while

I lift Jack out of the swing and bounce him on my hip. Bob waits kindly, but he looks skeptical about the likelihood that I'll be able to manage a newborn and run this magazine.

I am ready, Bob. I will not let you down.

Bob takes a weighted breath before continuing. "We need to increase our advertisers so we can go up to a forty-page book. We've printed thirty-two pages, which is okay, but doesn't look as professional as forty or forty-eight pages."

Laiah flashes past ready to launch her work day. She looks sleek in a business pantsuit. Her hair is styled, but not too flashy. No post-pregnancy blotchiness on her flawless skin. Laiah is the professional woman who should be at this meeting in my place. I situate Jack back in his swing, sit at the table, and open my notebook. "Now that the kids are back in school, I'll be heading down to Goodyear to talk with everyone. I really think everyone will keep advertising. They've been happy so far."

"Well, sometimes that summer break gives people an excuse to back out. I hate to go so long without talking to my clients in person."

Lowering my eyes, I turn away from Laiah so that Aaron and Bob won't notice her and compare her against me. She hounded me every day over the summer to get Jack's birth announcement written and mailed to my advertising customers. It had been on my to-do list and I'm ashamed I didn't get it done. There is an awkward silence. My voice is compensatory. "I'm confident my advertisers will continue." I try to reassure Bob that I won't ruin his magazine or his credibility.

At the front door, Bob rubs the back of his neck. "Okay, well, we only have two weeks until deadline. I wish we were further along"—he looks conflicted about what he's said; his marriage to LuDene is a second marriage for them both—"but I know you needed to go see your family and let them meet Jack. I'm glad you had a good vacation."

When talking about our summer, people keep using the word *vacation*. "A four-week vacation? How lucky." It sounds gluttonous, but if I've just had a four-week vacation, why am I *exhausted?* My body wants to crawl back into bed and take that nap Annice offered me after Jack was born.

Closing the door behind Bob, I want to sink down to the floor and cry. Aaron has gone back to the office. As far as he's concerned the magazine is doing fine. Apparently the pressure of acquiring eight new pages of advertising is only weighing on me. Not once during our meeting did Bob ask Aaron how many new accounts he intends to sell, nor did Aaron mention his plans to bring in new advertisers. Wasn't that our deal all along? I would get us started, but when Aaron resigned, he would take over the advertising sales. Of the two of us, he's the more experienced salesperson and I have an infant to feed every three hours.

Somehow, none of that came up in the conversation.

Heading to the office, I run into Laiah around the corner. She must know what I'm about to do. "Don't ask Aaron for help. It doesn't count if you have to ask for it."

In the office I slide my chair next to Aaron. "Look how cool this is." He shows me his design for a new business logo. He doesn't seem at all stressed by our pending print deadline.

I phrase my words carefully. "Aaron, I wanted to get down to Goodyear today to contact our advertisers, but the meeting lasted two hours. Between feeding Jack, drive time, and getting back for piano, I'd only have thirty minutes down there."

Aaron experiments with different color schemes for the logo.

"Tomorrow the kids have dentist appointments that have been scheduled for six months and it's Jack's two-month checkup." This reminds me that I need to schedule my six-week postpartum visit. I'm several weeks past due and the episiotomy hasn't healed. "Waiting until Wednesday will be too long…"

"I can go this afternoon," Aaron offers. "Are there certain people you want me to contact?"

Tanner comes in from the garage and launches his empty sippy cup at me. That means he wants more water. "Dawg, dawg?" He pats his mouth saying he's hungry for a hot dog. *Should I fix lunch for Tanner or prepare a contact list for Aaron?* My priorities are so confused. I pause, hoping Aaron will volunteer to feed Tanner, but he turns back to his computer.

"Let me go through my notes and make a list," I tell Aaron, then I turn to Tanner. "Go find your firetruck and play a little longer." I put the sippy cup out of sight hoping he'll forget, then plop down in a chair and lift out the portable file box from beneath my desk. This file is where I keep ad samples, business cards, and pending sales. The file box is dusty. I pull the names of a few of my most reliable customers for Aaron. "These are copies of the ad they ran last issue. Ask if they want to change their sales promotion or keep the same ad. And be sure to tell Randy that I said hello."

After lunch Aaron leaves. Tanner brings a book and cuddles up next to me on the couch while Jack nurses. My free arm pulls him close. The book is one of Tanner's favorites, *Ten Apples Up on Top*. He loves watching the characters stack more and more apples on their heads trying to outdo each other. "Apples, apples up on top. All of this must stop, stop, STOP!" Tanner leans his head into my shoulder. "Oh no, all our apples are going to drop."

He knows what's going to happen when I turn the page. He pulls his fingers out of his mouth long enough to say, "Cwash." Tanner looks at the illustration of apples flying across the page. "Uh-oh." He points.

"Crash! Uh-oh is right. What a big mess." I stroke Tanner's cheek watching the flutter of his lashes as his eyes close. My eyes beg to close, too, but I need to dig out the music and lesson plans from the Tucson conference. Where did Aaron put it all? Plus, Carol is on the piano lineup today and she can't see my house like this. She once told me when her son was young, she vacuumed her house twice a day because little kids spend so much time on the floor. My carpet hasn't been vacuumed for two months. It was fine for Bob, but I'm skeptical my blatant act of carpet neglect will escape Carol's scrutiny.

Mondays are my longest teaching days starting with my adult students. Linda arrives first, setting her cane inside the door and stepping in with a limp. "How is the family adjusting to the new baby?" She settles herself on the bench, opens her music bag, and hands me a container of state quarters for the kids' collection. She spent her summer home, in Pennsylvania, and stocks us with P-stamped quarters. Out west we get the Denver mint in circulation.

Next is Rachel, a reporter for the *Surprise Independent*. Her news story about my first piano recital filled my teaching slots and she became a student herself. Rachel's lessons are always filled with juicy tidbits of local gossip. We are twin sisters living mirror opposite lives. She sits on the bench envisioning her life with a husband and children. I sit on my chair imagining my life as a single woman reporting the daily news. We bond over the stress of print deadlines.

At 2:15 I see Carol's eyes scan my floor for fresh vacuum lines in the carpet. She presents me with a piece of pottery courtesy of her husband's latest hobby. "Thank you" is all I say, not sure whether to call it a candlestick or a goblet.

At 2:40 the carpool delivers Danny and Kate, who burst through the front door carrying the energy of a school ground. The commotion is impossible to ignore. Carol stops playing and smiles while they run to me and empty the contents of their backpacks at my feet. "Hi guys. How was your first day?" I let them hug me, but for Carol's sake, I have to interrupt their simultaneous chatter. "I'm teaching now, you can tell me all of this later. Go wash your hands and start your homework." Carol's eyebrows raise. Laiah would tell me that she's wondering why my children aren't better trained.

Mrs. O'Riley stays to observe Mallory's lesson. "May I use your bathroom?" she requests. She wears horn-rimmed reading glasses on a chain around her neck, reminiscent of a 1960s school librarian. I point the way down the hall and hope that Danny's after-school aim was on target and that Kate remembered to flush her number two. Mallory is learning middle D position with Mrs. O'Riley knitting furiously in the background when Kate marches in. With all the authority of an almost-six-year-old girl, she announces, "Jack has poop everywhere and it's disgusting."

Ethan takes Mallory's place on the bench while I power-wash the diaper disaster. Chrissy arrives early on purpose so she can play with our set of rescue hero toys. Once my last student leaves, I lean against the door. Four hours of clapping in rhythm to *Hot Cross Buns* and my head is a ticking metronome.

Jack fell asleep to his swing's rocking motion after his diaper change. "Let's get some food into your tummy, little man." Negotiation with Danny is required before I can claim ownership of the remote control. The art of diplomacy. Who says I'm not using my political science degree? Aaron walks in precisely three minutes later to see me with feet propped up watching the last five minutes of *Oprah*. For years this is what my life has looked like to him: reclining on a couch all day watching television. I can hardly wait for him to get a taste of what this "staying home" business is really about.

Aaron unloads groceries. My budget antennae is on high alert as I catalogue the items he sets on the counter. Every duplicate is money down the drain. "How much did you spend?"

Aaron doesn't know how much he spent. He digs in a bag for the receipt. When I shop, I know my total within fifty cents before getting to the checkout line because I've been adding the sum as I go, removing non-essentials if the tally gets too high. Aaron doesn't even compare prices. "Next time you're going, let me know and I'll send you with coupons."

"I wasn't planning to go, but I knew we needed food. I didn't know if you had anything planned for dinner."

The fact that he assumes nothing is planned for dinner vexes me. Danny reads his homework to me. I rub at a scabby, dry spot of skin beneath my left earlobe until the raw skin oozes with clear liquid. Jack eats, Danny reads, and I feel guilty about Aaron cooking dinner.

The whole situation is annoying.

But Aaron was right.

I didn't have anything planned for dinner.

———

ONCE DINNER IS over and the kids are tucked in, I spread a blanket on the office floor and let Jack play on his tummy so I can talk to Aaron. "How did the sales contacting go today? Were you able to talk to anyone?"

"Yes. Randy said to tell you hello. They aren't going to run an ad this month."

The weight of a bowling ball drops into my stomach. "You're kidding." Randy's full-color ad is my third-highest revenue. "Was his wife there with him?"

"Yes."

"You never ask about the ad when Verna is there. She micromanages the business funds. If Verna is there, you talk about her poodle and leave." Maybe I can catch Randy alone when I go out Wednesday and he'll change his mind. It terrifies me to ask about the rest of his afternoon.

"Phil and Amy at the framing shop are in the process of selling, so they aren't going to run. They said to contact the new owners in October."

"Did you tell them that if they run continuously, the new owners can keep the same rate instead of coming in at the higher rate?"

"No."

"Did you offer to design a new ad introducing the new owners? Maybe the new owners would pay for that. It would be good publicity."

"No. They said they didn't want to run, so I didn't force the issue." He turns back to his screen; I turn to my desk.

Did he do anything *to save that ad?* From January to April I'd spent hours stopping in and chatting with Phil before he finally agreed to *try* an ad. When several customers brought in the coupon from our magazine, he was ecstatic, saying it was the most effective advertising he'd ever done. Did Aaron remind him of any of that? No, because Aaron doesn't know about Phil's coupons. Aaron doesn't know about Verna or her poodle. Phil and Amy were my most reliable advertisers. The first day out and two ads down already. Hunched over my keyboard, I lean my forehead in my hands and fret about how to recoup the damage. Aaron powers off his computer, says goodnight, and steps over Jack. He leaves me staring at a towering stack of mail, the heaviness of my to-do list threatening to crush me.

Laiah enters quietly. You'd never guess that she's been through a full day of work: The front pleat of her pantsuit still looks freshly ironed, not a strand of her hair is out of place. "There are leftover tacos in the kitchen," I tell her. My stomach growls; I could eat a seven-course horse, but there's so much to do. Laiah chooses not to eat; instead she sits close and works with me, sifting through the mound of papers.

She sorts the grocery ads. "Cream of chicken soup is on sale."

On a scrap paper I scrawl a tentative meal plan, but a few months away from my own kitchen and it's as if I've forgotten how to cook. I can't create a single menu.

"Here's a coupon for fifty cents off tuna fish." Laiah insists on cutting and keeping the coupon, though my family detests tuna.

Moving to the mail, she rips open envelopes and directs my attention to the contents. Metropolitan Life encourages me to request a quote for life insurance. Del Webb Hospital provides instructions to obtain Jack's official birth certificate. Progressive asks if I'm paying too much for car insurance. I pause. *Am I paying too much for car insurance?* The letter gets stacked in a priority to-do pile. My desk is so messy it's almost polluted; a gray smog settles in the office choking my lungs. Laiah uncovers a sticky note reminding me in capital letters: *SCHEDULE 6 WEEK POSTPARTUM CHECKUP*. Jack stirs, flipping his head side to side, sucking on each fist, hoping one will produce milk. But we keep our noses pointed at task hoping that if we keep digging, we'll eventually find my brain in the pile.

Sometime later, Laiah and I finally stop talking. Three Boston Marathons have happened since waking this morning. Climbing into bed, my body sighs with the reprieve of being horizontal. I slide my feet back and forth between the comfort of the sheets. Over the summer we'd watched that movie about the endurance horse race across the Arabian Desert where Viggo Mortensen and his horse eat locusts, their only sustenance to get them through the arduous journey. This has been the longest day. In a few hours Jack will wake me, and tomorrow I get to repeat it all again.

CHAPTER 23

Circus

WEDNESDAY MORNING AARON pounds his alarm, sits partway up, and collapses against the headboard. I crack open one eye and check on Jack who is sleeping between us. Aaron's hair is smashed flat on one side and poking out wildly on the other. He looks like he's come from battle. "Who invited Barnum and Bailey's here last night?"

Throughout the night Danny, Tanner, and Jack took turns rotating through our bedroom like three performing bears on unicycles—Danny complaining about Tanner kicking him, Tanner begging to "sweep in my cwib, pwease," and between those two, Jack's unignorable wail. From midnight to 5:00, Aaron and I volleyed turns as ringmasters of the greatest spectacle on earth.

Now at 5:30 a.m. the house is peacefully quiet, no signs of the rumble that took place in the night. Aaron punches his pillow. "I cannot do any more nights like last night." He takes a four-minute shower and leaves for seminary. This year he is the seminary supervisor, which means he doesn't have to teach every day, but he's there several days a week and substitutes often.

My intent is to get up and shower, but I drift back to sleep. When Aaron closes the garage door, I sit up in panic. "Can you get Danny and Kate to school this morning so I can get ready to leave for Goodyear?"

Aaron pulls off his tie. "I have an appointment at 8:30 with the city planner."

"Why?"

"Remember that business idea I told you about, the education program for migrant workers? I stopped by the city offices Monday and talked with the mayor for over an hour. She loves the idea."

When did he have time Monday to talk to the mayor for over an hour? When I thought he was contacting advertisers? When he could have been home managing the kids during piano lessons? "You knew this morning would be my first chance to visit my customers. I told you on Monday." My voice grows louder, and Jack wakes up crying. I lift up my pajama shirt and let him latch on. "Did you make any contacts for the magazine yesterday while I was at the dentist with the kids?"

"Yes." Aaron's tone is indignant. "I handed out about twenty flyers." He huffs into the bathroom slamming the door shut. I walk into Kate's room with Jack attached to my chest and nudge her with my foot. "Wake up. Time to get ready for school." Still feeding Jack, I spread butter on toast and fill juice cups.

When Aaron leaves for the mayor's office and Tanner is engaged in *Barney's Good Manners*, I sit in the office pounding my fist against my forehead, trying to shake loose a clue about which task is most important. My cursor flits over the computer screen ultimately clicking the Photoshop icon. I've been trying to teach myself Photoshop so that I can stay home and do the design and layout work while caring for Jack, and Aaron can go out selling. Technology and I have an unstable relationship; neither of us quite knows how to handle the other. The tools and symbols of Photoshop seem a foreign language. Following a tutorial, I open a picture of my oldest brother and practice cropping out and attaching his face to different bodies. In October, Karl will be the first of my siblings to turn forty years old and I'm working on a funny cover for his birthday card.

When Laiah comes in, she asks, "What is that you're goofing around with?"

"I'm learning design," I justify the time-wasting. "You've got to see these." My mouse clicks and the folder of photos I created for Karl's fortieth birthday opens.

Laiah laughs at the images of Karl's head superimposed as Mr. Rogers, as captain of the *Starship Enterprise*, and as a dancing John Travolta. "You're getting really good with Photoshop."

AARON RETURNS AND I click off the monitor so he can't see how I've spent my morning hours. He hands me the car keys and I give him a list of instructions. "Jack went down for a nap at 10:00. He should wake up to eat at noon. I pumped and there's a bottle in the fridge. Don't let Tanner fall asleep before 1:00 or he'll be awake during piano lessons." Aaron mumbles an okay. I don't ask how the meeting went with the city planner. I don't care. Today my focus has to be recovering the lost ads.

PHIL IS IN the workroom of his frame store assembling the matting on a bridal portrait. His clerk shows me to the back. "That's gorgeous." I rave how the colors of the matting compliment the photo's composition. He places the four sides of the frame to let me glimpse the final result.

"The frame is the perfect selection of elegance and simplicity. You do beautiful work."

Phil looks pleased. We trade family stories. He asks about the baby. I wish him luck on his upcoming move. When all is said and done he loves the idea of running an ad and splitting the cost with the new owners.

Leaving Phil's shop, I race to catch Randy before he leaves for lunch. It's Wednesday and Verna will be gone to her pinochle game. The building is a huge warehouse-turned-discount furniture store. My dress heels click across the concrete floor. Randy is behind his desk checking a price for a customer who is tapping her foot. I recognize her.

"Cynthia Moake?" I hold out my hand. "I'm Maleah Warner. I bought your house on Memory Lane."

Cynthia looks confused, like she can't place my face. Dressed for business, I don't look the part of stay-at-home mother she met four years ago when I pushed Danny and Kate in a stroller up the sidewalk and knocked on the door asking about her house.

"I've never been able to tell you how much we love your house. You thought of so many great details. We love the air conditioned, carpeted garage. I taught dance classes there and my kids use it as a playroom."

At last it seems Cynthia makes the connection that I am the young mom who moved into her pristine house with a couple of sticky children. My intent was to thank her for the beautiful house, but she immediately makes apologies. "I'm so sorry I didn't paint the walls before I left. I never meant to leave them plain white." And "Oh my goodness, I'm such a mess today. I've been sewing and painting all morning."

Randy keeps his finger holding the place in the catalogue and listens while Cynthia tells me about a huge, empty home she's furnishing in Litchfield Park.

"My magazine mails to Litchfield Park. Have you seen it?" I show her my June copy opened to Randy's ad on the inside front cover.

"This is yours? I get it in the mail."

Randy's face perks up.

Sometime later, I leave Heartland Furniture with Randy's signature renewing his full-season contract. How could he not? My publication brought in Cynthia Moake, the TV-appearing, upscale, professional interior designer, who a few minutes earlier probably wrote him a check for ten times the cost of his ad for the year. We didn't mention his conversation with Aaron about discontinuing.

Thank you, Cynthia.

Aaron might consider spending my entire morning working two accounts to be an abhorrent waste of time. This work is neither speedy nor efficient. Kind of like mothering.

WHEN I GET home, Aaron is kneeling outside Danny and Tanner's bedroom with a screwdriver, reversing the door handles so the locks are on the outside. He has taken apart Jack's crib, moved it out of their room, and reassembled it in the corner of our bedroom.

For the next several nights after being tucked in, Tanner climbs out of bed and tries the door handle. We ignore his knocking. Eventually Tanner gives up and climbs back into bed. A couple of mornings we find that Tanner has slept on the floor by the door all night. When Danny complains about Tanner keeping him awake I say, "You don't have to sleep by Tanner. You can sleep out on the back porch." Danny chooses Tanner over the back porch.

I've found *the back porch* to be a universal cure for myriad parenting dilemma:

"You can eat your peas or you can go sit on the back porch."

"You can practice the piano or you can clean the back porch."

If the back porch isn't enough, I add the front porch for more effect: "If I hear one more sound from this bedroom, one of you will be sleeping on the back porch and one of you will be sleeping on the front porch. And it is raining."

That night Aaron and I pinky promise not to get up with Jack, but to let him cry himself back to sleep. At 2:00 a.m. we are wide awake listening to Jack's third bawling session of the night. My engorged breasts are virtually spraying milk like Yellowstone geysers in response to his cries. This is my fourth set of breast pads, but pumping will only train my body to continue producing milk at midnight. At last I kick off the covers. "I'm going to feed him."

Aaron protests. "He's old enough to get through the night without eating."

"He's going to wake up every hour until morning. I need sleep!" I try to sit on the loveseat to nurse, but my head keeps bobbing and I'm afraid of dropping Jack, so I bring him into bed with me and let him stay there until morning.

"He's not going to sleep through the night if you keep bringing him to bed with us," Aaron says the next morning.

Three and a half hours of sleep was not enough. I can hardly get my body into the shower. Today is morning appointments in Goodyear followed by another afternoon of piano lessons. Bending to shave, I feel a pain shoot down my leg. The episiotomy. Today I *have* to remember to call and schedule my postpartum checkup.

CHAPTER 24

Postpartum Visit

THE NEXT WEEK I shake Danny's shoulder. "Hey bud. Wake up. You have to get ready super fast. We all slept late." Danny pulls the covers close to his chin. "Danny!" I yank the covers off and lift him out of bed onto his feet. He wobbles on unsteady legs. "Can you get dressed by yourself, please? I have to shower and get myself ready." My six-week postpartum checkup is today, *finally*, though I gave birth nine weeks ago. Danny drops back onto his bed. I heft his weight and maneuver him to the bathroom standing him on my feet in front of the toilet. The whoosh of urine splashes around the porcelain bowl, spraying the floor and my bare feet. With one arm I balance him upright—he sways like a drunk man—and with the other hand I wipe the drips. Once he's dressed, I repeat the same process with his sister. These are the same kids who were awake by sunrise every morning this summer?

Our shower has to run twenty minutes before the water turns warm. We live in the hottest state in America and can't get a hot shower. There's no time to wait; I wash in frigid water. *You have so much to do!* I chastise myself for sleeping late. Out of the shower I pump a bottle of milk for Jack.

"Hurry, get your backpack!" I shoo Danny away from his bed where he was recounting for Tanner how Pikachu evolves from Pichu then into Raichu. I don't understand Pokémon, but Danny seems to have memorized every Pokémon's region, type, energy, and weakness. He should have no problem mastering the Periodic Table of Elements. Down the hall Kate is slumped onto the floor next to her bed singing to the socks she dangles before her face. I grab the socks out of her hand and hastily slide them onto her feet.

"Ouch!" she complains.

"If you had done it yourself, then it wouldn't hurt! Get your backpack and meet me in the car!"

Rushing out the front door, I see Danny and Kate twirling on the front lawn. "Get in the car. Get in the car!" I shout.

They stop spinning and stare.

"Don't stand there. Get. In. The. Car!"

"Your car or Dad's car?" Kate asks.

Now *I* stop, uncertain. Which keys did I grab? Do I need the vehicle with the car seats today or does Aaron? We don't know whose car is whose anymore. We're always juggling who has the keys or the kids, who is staying home and who is leaving. We either schedule conflicting appointments or we're home at the same time—this is when we butt heads.

Our kids are even more off kilter. Dad is working from home now, but he's still working and they aren't accustomed to asking him for help. I'm home, but not necessarily *here*.

I look at the keys in my hand. "Get in the van."

On the drive to school Danny asks, "Mom, why are you going to the doctor? Are you going to get another baby out?" I said that we already had a little baby and did he think we needed another? He contemplated the issue seriously then nodded. "I'd like twenty-five babies."

"Yeah!" Kate bounces with enthusiastic agreement.

Twenty-five babies! Heaven help us.

THE NURSE AT Dr. Woods' office hands me a paper exam gown. My legs poking out from under the cherry-red paper look like the two wooden handles of a popsicle. Overhead the air conditioner blows chilled air directly on me. Outside it's 106 degrees, but lying on this exam bed I might as well be sitting on a shelf in the freezer. Goosebumps speckle my pasty skin. The bright medical lights overhead bring back blurry memories of Jack's birth. Being here at this hospital for the first time since the delivery summons a deluge of emotions and again—as happens any time I recall that night—I'm flooded with regret.

So many questions, I don't know which to ask first. Aaron wants me to mention *it* to Dr. Woods, but I don't feel depressed. Something doesn't feel right with me, but *it* is not depression.

When Dr. Woods comes in, I can tell he is rushed for time. "Hello," he says with a warm smile, washing his hands. "How old is baby? Nine weeks already?" He opens my gown for a breast examination. "Sorry if my hands are cold." He moves down the table to extend the stirrups. "You know, sometime I'd like to actually deliver one of your babies." Dr. Woods laughs as he reaches for a speculum.

"I'm sorry." I apologize with genuine guilt. "I tried to hold on. Really, I did."

"Ooh, that looks tender." Dr. Woods wrinkles his brow as he examines my episiotomy. "Which doctor delivered you?"

"It was the on-call doctor, Dr. Babich." My biggest regret was not being delivered by Dr. Woods. He wasn't there and I'd been manhandled by a strange doctor who'd stitched me like a ripped canvas tent. This summer I'd driven too many hours on the horrid episiotomy. "Will I always have an extra hole down there?" I wince as he probes the crooked seam.

"We can re-stitch it if we need to, but it looks like it will close on its own."

All the emotions of the past nine weeks surge up—the words are practically fighting to get out of my throat. My heart pounds in urgent need to sit up and blurt the whole story to Dr. Woods: the road to Tucson, my dilemma about when to go to the hospital, how I'd held on so he could deliver me, how I was here on that

Monday—did he remember turning me away?—then the bath, the Tylenol PM, the speed of the delivery. There is so much I want to do over, which doesn't make sense to Aaron, but it will make sense to Dr. Woods. I'm too close to the situation to know if it's real or all in my head, but this wise doctor will make *it* all better. This has been my hope and prayer for the appointment—that Dr. Woods will know how to fix me.

My lungs need a refill of air and then I'm ready to start pouring out my heart, but Dr. Woods slides the stool back and rips off his latex gloves. "If the episiotomy hasn't healed in a few weeks, come back in. Otherwise, everything looks good. Congratulations on the baby."

But…

Aaron made me promise.

"Um, wait…I do have one question."

He stops with one hand on the doorknob.

Another big breath. "Since Jack was born—no, well, just lately, maybe longer, I haven't been feeling well…" What specific symptoms could I give him? Nothing outside of being really stressed, moody, and completely disorganized, but a doctor can't fix that. "After my second baby…I think I might have had some postpartum depression…" Instantly I wish I could suck those words back in and swallow them down into the darkness of my bowels where they belong. "I mean, I don't know. I was never diagnosed…it went away on its own…"

Dr. Woods interjects. "Would you like a prescription for Wellbutrin?"

The room is silent, but inside my head is a buzz of questions:

What is Wellbutrin? Is it an antidepressant? How do you know if I need an antidepressant? Is it safe for breastfeeding? How do you know if I have postpartum depression? What if it's something bigger like a brain tumor? Do you test to see if a person's chemicals are out-of-balance before throwing in a complex drug with all its possible side effects? Do you have a list of questions I should answer before you prescribe medication? If

I start taking an antidepressant, will my body become dependent, so I have to take it for the rest of my life? What about my friend who had a horrible reaction to an antidepressant and ended up worse than before taking the medication? How do you know I won't be like her?

My brain can't form the swirl into coherent sentences. Beneath this paper gown I'm stark naked, my legs splayed out in stirrups—a frog on a dissection table—with jelly dripping down my inner thighs. My teeth chatter in the subarctic temperature. I want my clothes, my underwear, and my socks.

From my prostrate position, I crane my neck to see Dr. Woods at the door waiting on my answer; his next appointment is checking her watch in the neighboring room. He's my only doctor, but I'm not his only patient. While I have delivered four babies, he has delivered hundreds. He is special to me, but I am not unique to him. He sees dozens of pregnant women just like me, day after day, all year long. We stream in and out of his office like an assembly line of baby makers. To him I am routine.

My hope for this appointment was that he would take one look at me and immediately know what was wrong and how to fix it: "My dear! You have a foreign augmentative thoracic-cardiovascular neoplasm. Don't you worry. We'll have you fixed up in no time."

But Dr. Woods doesn't say that. I don't know what's wrong with me and apparently, he doesn't either.

"There are other medications like Zoloft, if you prefer," Dr. Woods offers.

I don't know any more about Zoloft than I do about Wellbutrin. My life is too complicated right now to make stab-in-the-dark guesses and play experimental prescription roulette. I can't afford to add one more unknown into the overcrowded chaos of my life. "No. No. No, but thank you. I think it's probably normal baby blues."

"Call our office if you change your mind." Dr. Woods makes a note on a paper and deposits my chart into the file holder on the door. I toss the used paper towels into the trash, peel off the gown, and stand bare-skinned in the middle of Dr. Woods' office, staring out the sixth-story window.

ON THE DRIVE home I recount the appointment for Laiah. The first tidbit she grasps onto is that Dr. Woods had made a note in my chart. Depression will be on my permanent record now. If anything mysterious happens to the kids, to Aaron, or to me, I will be the primary suspect because *it* is in my file. I ask Laiah if she thinks I made the right decision or if I should have taken the prescription.

Laiah says, "Every woman is tired and overwhelmed after having a baby. I don't think you have anything that's outside normal. It's not like you're going to drown your children. You're not Andrea Yates."

The thing that scares me about taking a drug, I tell her, is not knowing how the side effects will mess up my system. My family has crazy reactions to medications. I remember being fourteen years old and watching Annice nearly die from an allergic drug reaction after getting her wisdom teeth pulled. My brother went for a simple colonoscopy and ended up with an abdominal infection and three feet less colon than he started with. I've seen too many situations when drugs or medical intervention has made the patient worse than they were to begin with. True, I don't feel good, but I don't want to be worse.

Laiah agrees that taking medication isn't worth the risk, especially for something like *depression*, which is a mood disorder, not an illness. "Remember the interview with Dolly Parton on *Oprah*?" Laiah reminds me. "Dolly said that the best way to cure depression is to get off your butt and get to work."

I need to pull up my big girl bootstraps and adopt Dolly's no-nonsense attitude. Get up in the morning and exercise. Eat more nutritiously. Time and hard work are always the best medicines.

BEFORE SLEEP, I collapse on my knees against my bed. Tonight I mostly ask God to please help Jack sleep until morning. After my *amen* I crawl under the covers. Bed feels so good. Aaron rolls close, his hands slide up my pajama shirt. My body goes tense.

In the conversation about the episiotomy, Dr. Woods hadn't mentioned instructions about sex, and I'd forgotten to ask.

"It's been over two months." Aaron's hands freeze.

I don't know how to respond. No matter what I do, I can't win. Refuse and Aaron resents me. Consent and split a bigger opening, then will the episiotomy ever heal? My body has been probed, prodded, and excavated. My nipples have been sucked to ruination. I'm going to scream and pull out all my hair if one more person needs a piece of me! Go ahead, spread me out on a buffet table and devour away. I'm being eaten alive.

Aaron flips onto his back, his words aimed at the ceiling. "Did you ask Dr. Woods about postpartum depression?"

It takes me a *long* time to answer. His question grates at me. Is he implying that I'm avoiding sex because I'm *depressed?* I don't want to be in this bed with him. He has no idea what I'm going through. Why doesn't he hold me and say he's sorry that I'm split open in the crotch, that it must really hurt. Why doesn't he thank me for all my body has gone through to have our baby? He could say how amazing I am for everything I do during the day, despite being in pain. There are so many things he could say... Instead he points to another way he thinks I'm broken.

There is no way I can put all that into words. What comes out is simply, "I did."

"What did he say?"

"He asked if I wanted a prescription for Wellbutrin."

"Did you get the prescription?"

"No! He didn't do any tests."

"What tests are there?" Aaron asks.

"I don't know. But he didn't even ask questions."

"Don't you think you had *it* after Kate?"

"I don't know for sure. I don't know if there is a definitive test or if I was self-diagnosing. Besides, with Kate, *it* went away on its own."

Aaron is silent. He thinks *it* has never really gone away.

"I want to give it more time before trying drastic measures."

"Why is medicine a drastic measure?"

"I don't know anything about Wellbutrin. I don't know how my body will react."

"Did you ask?"

"We didn't really have time. I don't want to take a drug while I'm breastfeeding. And my body always reacts to medication differently than other people. It's normal for women to not feel right after having a baby."

Aaron rolls to the other side.

"We know more now. We know how to handle *it* better than we did before."

It.

That's how we refer to this thing neither of us can define nor describe—an unseen poltergeist that lives in the gutter. Every now and then we wake to the aftermath of its haunting, but can't exactly describe its face.

Aaron doesn't answer. An unmeasurable amount of time passes, thick with tension and mutual exhaustion, but devoid of sleep. Eventually Aaron's breath slows and deepens. Silently I wipe at my eyes with my pillowcase. Strange images from after Kate's birth pass through my head, but I don't dream.

CHAPTER 25

Episodes

MY EYES WATCH the ceiling fan make its rotation as the perplexing images from after Kate's birth pass through my mind like slides from ancient family vacations. Once again I wish I could convince myself these images are figments of hallucinations rather than snapshots of reality. It all seems to have happened so long ago, if it happened at all.

We were driving down Bell Road to a party at Annice's house with Danny and Kate buckled in the back seat. Danny, in full toddler vibrato, sang "Who Let the Dogs Out" while eighteen-month-old Kate joined in the chorus showcasing her newest animal sound: *woof*. From the outside, this polaroid looks every bit the happy family photo. Then, maybe Aaron asked a question about money, or perhaps his comment was as trivial as noticing the increase in traffic congestion with the snowbirds back in town. It could have been anything or nothing at all. My head was spinning (it had probably been spinning all morning). My chest tightened. My airway constricted. The car closed in on me. I couldn't tell Aaron what was wrong because I didn't know, I only knew that if I didn't get out of the car I was going to suffocate or burn.

At a red light, I opened my passenger door and walked in and out of four lanes of stopped cars. The light turned green before I stepped onto the curb. Horns honked angrily at Aaron, who was yelling for me to get back into the car. Without turning around, I crossed the parking lot and disappeared into a tobacco shop—a place Aaron would never look for me. It wasn't crowded in the tobacco shop; it was small, nowhere to hide, the clerk asked how he could help me today. I said never mind and went back outside.

After wandering the parking lot, I dropped down onto the curb, my feet in the gutter, head low like a homeless beggar. Aaron wouldn't call me—at the time neither of us had a cell phone. My feet kicked at gravel while I wondered if Aaron would turn around and go home, leaving me to figure my own way out of this. Maybe he would continue on to Annice's house, though it's awkward to arrive at your sister-in-law's house without her sister. He might come for me, and this is the scenario that played out in my mind, one train of thought anticipating him berating me harshly and the more wishful images of him running toward me, his eyes full of worry, scooping me in his arms, kissing my tears, and making *it* all better.

I hadn't even sat on the curb long enough for my capris to get dirty before the Taurus pulled up slowly and stopped in front of me. Aaron didn't get out, he just waited. Eventually I stood up, opened the door, and took my seat.

Aaron held tight to the steering wheel. "What on earth were you thinking?"

I hadn't been thinking. I didn't know *what* to think. When I'd opened the door, it was because I couldn't *be* in that place anymore, in that car, in my life, in that existence. I hadn't wanted to die. I'd only wanted to *get out*.

Aaron pulled out of the parking lot and continued to Annice's. "Tell me, what have I done to make your life so miserable? Is your life really that bad?"

I shook my head. My life wasn't bad. My life was incredibly good. I just wasn't cut out for it. Which made my self-hate more acrid.

By the time we arrived at Annice's house my face was cheerful, smiling, ready for the party. My red eyes were "these darned allergies." As the party progressed, I warmed up—talking, laughing, making jokes, and touching Aaron's arm with affection. And once we got back in the car for the drive home, the episode was gone, the flash of lightning disappeared. We didn't mention it. No reason to talk about a thunderstorm when the sun is shining.

MONTHS LATER HE found me sitting on the floor of the shower, water running over my head, comparing the blade of my razor to the large blue vein on the white skin of my wrist. I wanted him to see me. I had waited a long time, sitting in the shower with the water wasting, for him to come in from working in the yard. Jealous that the lawn and bushes got more attention from Aaron than me, I sat, wanting him to *see* me, wanting him to *rescue me*. When at last the bedroom door opened, I kept my head folded over my knees. Next the shower door opened in a fury, but he did not fall to his knees and scoop me up. Mixed with the rushing water, I heard his voice.

"Tell me!" he cried. "What do I do that makes you so miserable? Am I so hard to live with?" Then silence.

"It's not you," I finally yelled. "Just go! I'm not going to do anything." The blinds on our outside door rattled a long time after the door slammed. Against the tile wall, the razor shattered and bounced on the drain, the water pushing the plastic pieces like pebbles in a creek bed. I pounded my head against the back of the shower.

I don't remember getting out of the shower, but once I did, the rest of the day was laundry and Saturday chores, Aaron and I barely speaking to each other and certainly not mentioning *the incident*.

AT SOME POINT, Aaron and I began alluding to these outbursts (if we spoke of them at all) as *episodes*. This seemed the best term to describe my bizarre spurts of behavior, because they happened irregularly, came out of the blue, and seemed to turn on and off like a TV drama. Most often we sidestepped the topic, a couple of shell-shocked soldiers tiptoeing cautiously through a mine field.

Occasionally, during a tense conversation where one or neither of us were being careful, we said *it*.

Through trial and error (copious amounts of error), we figured out that *it*—whatever *it* was—raised *it*s monstrous head less often if I got out of the house by myself. We designated Thursdays as my night, and after dinner I left Aaron wrangling the kids and dishes and drove alone to the library. With unbridled rapaciousness, I cleared the periodical section of current issues and spent uninterrupted hours reading every cover article that had caught my attention in the grocery store checkout line. I did nothing but read until the librarian's voice on the intercom announced closing, and to please check out or return materials to their shelves. I never checked out books. With toddlers at home and a daily vocabulary maximum of two-syllable words, my brain didn't have the power to manage full-length novels. Each week I waited for the last possible second to re-shelve my stack of magazines and was the last person to exit the building, the librarian locking the door behind me. I went home feeling like an entirely new woman, more fortified to face my little nemesis for another seven days. Still, we watched nervously, Aaron and I, without speaking of *it*, for Mrs. Hyde to rupture.

For the most part after Tanner was born, all was calm. Aaron might disagree because there were still episodes, but for me there wasn't the constant undercurrent of blackness and despondency. The episodes were rare, smaller, certainly less frequent. I commented to other women how much more enjoyable the third baby is because you know what you're doing and can relax. During the time after Tanner's birth, we experienced a great deal of happiness (as well as a lot of noise) with our little family.

Sometime during all this, I heard an interview where Marie Osmond talked about driving away from home in the middle of the night. This was the first time I'd ever heard the term *postpartum depression*. After Kate's birth, when I drove away from home in the middle of the night headed toward Las Vegas to become a show girl,

I was convinced I was the only mother in the world who had ever done that. Marie's book came home with me from the library and I read it cover to cover. When I turned the final page, I felt better knowing there was at least one other woman on the planet who had taken her car keys in the middle of the night and driven away from home. Aaron still didn't know about my midnight escapade, but I commented to him about Marie's experience and this thing called postpartum depression. By this time, I was feeling better and any episodes were so random, unexpected, and spaced months in between, that *it* didn't seem to qualify as a permanent ailment. Without saying anything out loud, perhaps we both thought, "Hmm. Maybe there's something to that."

CHAPTER 26

Photoshop

OVER THE NEXT months I live a modified version of Newton's Law of Inertia, which goes something like this: A mother in motion must keep moving, because if she stops or sits down she will immediately fall asleep.

The September and October print deadlines come and go. My memory of those months consists of blurry images of Aaron or me pulling into our driveway and hastily exchanging keys for children—like the baton pass on a relay team. The new runner backs out and screeches down the road, leaving exhaust fumes and skid marks on the street called Memory Lane.

Now we are hustling to meet the November issue cutoff. The due date of October 17 looms over our house like a ponderous, dark task master. One might expect our organization and implementation to have significantly improved by this, our sixth publication deadline, but I'm questioning whether, come Monday, we'll have a magazine at all. The difference this month is that the kids have been out of school on a two-week fall break. My knees barely rolled under my desk the first day of school vacation when various tiny heads poked through the office door. "We want to go swimming. Can we ride our bikes to the park? We can't reach the finger paint. Will you help us build the train set?" For the rest of fall break, either I'm in the office feeling guilty that I should be spending time with the kids or I'm spending time with kids feeling guilty that I should be getting magazine work done in the office. I flit from one thing to another without finishing anything.

Kate was scheduled for a tonsillectomy over fall break at Del Webb Hospital, but the billing administrator called about a glitch with our insurance. Her surgery is indefinitely postponed while we file an appeal, because I need more paperwork like I need a root canal. Here I sit, trying to design an ad for Angel's Housecleaning Service. I met Angel at the Chamber of Commerce business breakfast. She is trying to build her clientele with no advertising budget, and I need a maid. Bob has agreed to let us trade an ad for bimonthly house cleaning.

In the afternoon, Laiah sits on my office desk flipping through pages of sample ads when she notices the name of a saved computer file. "What's this?" Laiah asks clicking a folder labeled *Maleah Before and After.*

"Oh, it's nothing." I say even though I know exactly what is in the file. Aaron had shown me, several nights ago, the new photo editing skills he'd learned from a Photoshop tutorial.

"Show me. I want to see." Laiah is curious.

"No time tonight. I need to focus and finish Angel's ad, then get the kids through the bath."

"It will only take a minute."

My mouse double clicks the file and the screen fills with side-by-side images of me cropped from a family photo. The photo has been zoomed in, magnifying my face from the neck up. Though both images are the exact same photo, there is a stark contrast between the woman on the left and the woman on the right.

"Wow, what tool did Aaron use to cover your pregnancy rash? You can't see it at all."

Clicking the history button, Laiah follows the step-by-step process required to erase my blotchy skin and remove the dark circles beneath my eyes. Aaron has thickened my eyelashes and defined my lips with an outline and color fill. In the second image my red acne bumps are gone. Laiah continues clicking, observing how magically the large mole on my neck disappears.

Staring at the differences between my own pocked face and the buttercream complexion of the Photoshopped version of me, it's impossible to ignore the many ways I fall short of perfection. The eyes of the woman in the improved photo stare at me. They are my eyes, but they aren't. My eyes are constantly streaked with red. This woman's eyes are white and clear. No sign of fatigue. Using skin filters, red-eye removal, teeth whitening, and blur tools, Aaron has used Photoshop to erase all my flaws. It's as if I'm seeing all the things Aaron would change about me if he were given a magic wand. If only it were so easy in real life.

I drag the Photoshop paintbrush tool over the images, scribbling red lines over both faces. Dropping my head into my hands, I close my eyes and rub my temples. *So much work to do. Focus!* But the walls of the office are closing in on me in the same way my ribs are crushing my lungs. Laiah shadows me as I flee the office followed by an ominous sense of déjà vu.

OPENING THE HEAVY sliding glass door to our backyard, I see the results of telling the kids to go outside to play. Kate and Tanner convinced Danny to pull the heavy garden hose into the sandbox and turn on the water for Mud Fun. I don't have the energy to wash them for dinner—their sand-coated legs and my white carpet are not a good combination—so I carry paper plates of spaghetti outside and they eat picnic-style on the grass. Rolling out a blanket on the grass for Jack consumes the rest of my strength; I collapse on my back next to him and watch as he kicks his feet and chews his hands while we gaze at birds in our palm trees. Jack is four months old. I never hold him, I juggle him. Thank goodness for breastfeeding or I might never pick him up. Lately Tanner has been acting up. He's starved for attention during the day because I only come out of the office long enough to slice his microwaved hot dog and lock him in his room for naptime without a story.

Tanner sneaks up behind Danny and dumps a bucket of wet sand over his head. The sun sets and I herd the trio out of the sandbox, strip them naked, spray them with the hose, and let them take their bath in the hot tub. Eventually there is more water on the patio than in the jacuzzi. "Time to get out." Kate does a power ranger spin move into the towel I'm holding, her foot slicing my arm and drawing blood. My hand grabs her ankle; her toenails are so long they could carve our Halloween jack-o-lanterns. "Run inside and get your pajamas on, all of you, then meet me on the couch for nail clipping." Their teachers must think they're neglected. Danny and Kate whoop and holler and race each other inside. Tanner toddles after, trying to keep up. His towel falls, the dimples in his full moon jiggle as he runs.

The jacuzzi cover feels heavier than normal. Usually a one-hand job, tonight it requires both my arms and a heave from my legs to lift, pull, unfold, and lock down the lid before lifting the wooden stairs on top. Our little garden hose resists my pulling and dragging; it feels as cumbersome, bulky, and awkward as a python.

In my bathroom I mean to fetch the nail clippers, but the wooden hamper box in my closet beckons me to sit down. The box is small, yet tonight its hard lid is inviting. I drop onto the seat and do nothing but sit. From the boy's room I hear that the mud-bathers have launched a jumping-on-the-bed tournament.

"What are you doing?" Aaron asks, coming in behind me.

"I don't know. I can't seem to move." I'm not injured. My body isn't broken or bleeding (other than the toenail gouging, courtesy of Kate), but standing requires a Herculean strength beyond my ability. My chest pounds with the *thump, thump* that our washing machine makes when it struggles to spin a load of beach towels. "I'm so tired." I want Aaron to say how I deserve to be tired, how I work myself to the bone, how he wishes I would slow down.

Instead he says, "Why?"

Silence is my response, so Aaron washes his hands and walks out of the bathroom.

Can't he *see* how exhausted I am? Turning around to the closet mirror, I expect to see the skeletal shadow of a sickly woman—that's how I feel—and I wonder how Aaron could walk past so unfeelingly when I'm on the brink of collapse. Instead, the woman in the mirror looks like the normal me with acne bumps, pregnancy rash, and red eyes—somewhat unkempt, but certainly not appearing to need medical attention.

The sound of Aaron's steps goes straight back to the office, walking past the kids' bedroom, doing nothing about the full-out brawl happening within. From the opening and closing of doors, I can tell that Kate is bringing pillows from her room. In frustration, I fling the nail clippers at the bathroom wall and fold in half, putting my face between my legs and using my knees to tighten the grip of my hands squeezing my head, trying to hold it all together.

A loud *thunk!* from the bedroom brings me back to reality. The kids are pushing the mattress off the bed preparing to make a super-slide. Mustering strength from somewhere, I lift my body off the hamper box and go to assess the damage. The kids are all stark naked, launching themselves off the bed onto pillows they've gathered from every room. I clap my hands and shout orders to get pajamas on, teeth brushed and go straight to bed. Three bare bodies run past me for the bathroom. My shoulder pushes the mattress onto its box spring. The sheets have to be re-tucked. Passing the office, I see Aaron sorting through the mounds of mail on my desk.

"Isn't sorting the mail your thing?" Laiah tags along.

The kitchen becomes a studio of bangs, clanks, and crashes. Toys tossed in the cupboards, plates loaded in the dishwasher, the growl of the vacuum, water running for mopping. "Don't come out here," I call down the hall to Aaron, "the floor will be wet." I hear a light "Okay" from the office.

Once the mop is rung out, my feet slide on paper towels down the hall to the office. While the floor dries, I can finally show Aaron the draw-up for a new salon ad. My computer screen has just woken up when Aaron clicks off his computer.

"Goodnight." He walks past, not stopping to kiss me.

"Is he mad at you tonight?" Laiah asks.

"I don't know. I think he's frustrated with me. He's always following me, cleaning up the messes I leave, doing the things I haven't gotten around to. It annoys him that I'm always running behind."

"He doesn't look at you the way he used to in college."

When we were engaged, Aaron acted like he'd won the future wife jackpot, but it didn't take long for him to discover he'd gotten a lemon. Laiah and I often question if he stays with me out of duty. If he weren't a religious man, bound by the covenant of marriage, would he trade me in for a better model?

With Aaron off to bed, I work on the ad myself, but my brain is fuzzy. After twenty minutes, I have a rectangle and a few wavy lines. Laiah peers over my shoulder. "Aaron would have finished this ad by now and it would look a lot more professional than that."

I kick my chair away from the desk and pound my head.

"Are you quitting?" Laiah asks. "I thought you wanted to learn ad design so you could take over and Aaron could do sales."

Suddenly the screen goes blank, a pop-up window appears: *Photoshop shut down unexpectedly. Unsaved changes lost. Report problem?* I click *Don't Report* and shut down the computer. In the kitchen I crawl on my hands and knees with a rag and cleaner, polishing the floor to a sheen. But no matter how hard I rub, I can't seem to erase the barrage of photoshopped images in my head, the evidence of all the ways I don't measure up.

While Jack eats, I click through late night TV shows hoping the sound will drown out the maddening storm in my mind. There's an ants-in-the-pants feeling under my skin keeping me from getting comfortable. I can hardly wait for Jack to finish so I can put him back to bed. I'm not myself tonight, I'm a woman from five years ago, a woman I hoped to never encounter again.

Opening the door to our bedroom, I'm surprised to see Aaron wide awake reading a book. I get ready for bed and pull up the covers. The fall air is thick with heat, but even though Aaron has kicked his portion of the comforter onto my side of the bed doubly insulating me, I can't stop shaking. I tighten my muscles to keep the convulsions from disturbing Aaron. It isn't exactly like being cold, it's more like being absent of heat. Something in me is missing and all I can do is shake for the emptiness.

Hadn't we figured this out already? Hadn't I nipped *it*? Not only am I getting out once a week, I am *working*. I dress up in business attire with styled hair and makeup and speak with adults. Each month a paycheck arrives with *my* name on the payee line. The question of whether I possess brains or ability to run a business has been settled; my *savoir faire* has been proven, has it not? One could argue that when it comes to advertising sales, I have outperformed Aaron. Wasn't it being stuck at home that had driven me crazy after Kate?

The shaking escalates. I'm an Eskimo in an earthquake. Staying in bed is not an option. I can't be next to Aaron. Out of bed I realize that I can't stay here in this bedroom. I can't *be* anywhere, not in this house, not in this existence. My life doesn't fit anymore, like I've put two legs into one pant leg and can't move forward until it's fixed. I don't know where to go; I only know that I cannot stay.

Aaron sits up watching me tie the laces on the running shoes I've brought out from the closet. "Please don't leave."

We have learned by hard experience how *not* to deal with these episodes, so we talk for a while. *Do you need to get out more?* he asks. *I'm out of the house every day*, I answer, *I just don't feel good.*

Tonight, talking doesn't help.

I'm a ticking time bomb and neither of us knows how to disable me.

"I have to go. I know you want to help, but we both know you can't and staying here only makes me more frustrated."

Aaron's face asks a thousand silent questions. He witnesses me lifting the car keys from the dresser, neither blind nor resistant to the sequence of events; his eyes show plain enough that he doesn't like the situation—doesn't like me leaving, doesn't like not having the answer that fixes everything—but what surprises me most is that he lets me go, and that I let him.

My neighborhood is quiet. Rolling gray clouds move in front of the moon. My body is trembling as I start the ignition and back out of the driveway. This is not a *Thelma & Louise* copycat game. In my core there is no desire to drive off a cliff or crash into a barrier going ninety miles per hour. Though my chest houses an explosive device, my mind remains connected to at least one thread of control. This is not a prison break, an escape from my life. This is a search to find how to remove the ticking bomb without detonating me in the process. *Can someone please show me how to* be *in my life?*

Each turn of the steering wheel is an evaluation of my options. The emergency room? No, they will pump me full of drugs, lock me away, take my children. I don't want to be numbed, to become a drug-altered version of me. The police station? No. The police would have to notify child protective services. Another option is to drive for a while, hoping the fuse on the dynamite peters out. I need help. This is not me driving away from help, this is me driving toward help.

But where to go?

I need somewhere safe. I need to talk with someone who is neutral and nonjudgmental, someone who isn't perfect—no, someone who isn't afraid of being *seen* as imperfect. I need someone who has a messy, chaotic, mistake-filled life and who is okay with people knowing that.

I need Amanda.

CHAPTER 27

Midnight Visit

AMANDA USED TO teach Sunday School at church. She made the New Testament real and applicable in today's world, as if Jesus and the disciples could stop by Burger King and pick up a Whopper on their way to the Sea of Galilee, except on Fridays when they would order a fish sandwich. Amanda wasn't afraid to be flawed. While the rest of us sat properly dressed in our Sunday best with pasted-on smiles, Amanda told stories about blowing up and launching a garbage can at her husband.

One Friday I'd invited Amanda and Derek for a couples' dinner and game night at our house. About the time we expected them to ring our doorbell, she telephoned to say they wouldn't be coming because she and Derek were in the middle of having "the war of the century"—her words exactly. I felt embarrassed that, in a moment of weakness, she'd spilled a secret about her marriage she would regret later. At church the next Sunday, I expected her to avoid me out of shame, but she walked right up and poured her friendly, nonjudgmental "Hello" all over me.

Several years ago, she and Derek moved into a new house and started going to a church building closer to their new neighborhood. Considering my lack of geographical sense combined with the fact that I've only been to her new house once before, it's nothing short of miraculous that I drive straight here. Her house is completely dark. The entire street is silent—no stray dogs, no cars, no teenagers hanging on the corner. I question my decision to come. We don't have what you'd call a "knock once and come on in" relationship, especially after midnight. Turning off my headlights, I realize it's been several years since I've spoken to her. Maybe she won't remember me.

"You're where?" Laiah asks when I call. "She's going to think you're certified crazy."

My mother raised eight kids, ran a farm, bottled her own fruit, and never cried a day in her life. How did I end up parked in someone's driveway after midnight wearing pajamas?

"What are you going to do? Ring the doorbell?" Laiah asks. "And what will you say, 'Hi, Amanda, I happened to be in the neighborhood, so I thought I'd stop by?'"

I climb out of the car and shut my door as quietly as possible, even though I'm planning to ring the bell and wake them up. No sane person would knock on someone's door this late, but as confused as my mind tends to be, I feel absolute certainty I'm in the right place.

My first knock is soft. Hopefully Amanda is a light sleeper. Maybe she'll happen to be walking by the front door just now.

No one answers.

The next knock is a bit louder.

My finger starts to compress the doorbell button, then I pull back anticipating how loud the bell will echo in the solitude. I imagine lights flicking on in surrounding houses, dogs barking, men appearing on their lit doorstops with shotguns and Amanda having to come out and apologize to her neighbors for the disturbance from her "special" friend. As much as I want to, as much as I need to, I can't ring the doorbell. The tips of my tennis shoes rock up and down on the front step and look oddly out of place with my pajamas, the same way I look oddly out of place hovering at a door in the middle of the night.

So, to the emergency room?

I'm turning to leave when I hear a voice coming from above and behind me.

"Who are you?" the voice asks. A man's head looms in the darkness about ten feet to my left, lit aglow from a streetlamp. Unblinking eyes bore into me. "What are you doing?" the head asks.

It takes a moment to get my bearings and realize that Amanda's neighbor is looking over his fence, which is tall enough that only his head shows above it.

"Um, I was just…I mean…"

My desperation must show on my face because the man says, "Are you okay?" The head turns to take a puff from a cigarette. This complete stranger perceives what those close to me miss: that I am not well.

"I was coming to see Amanda, but it looks like they are all asleep, so I'll come back another time." My feet shuffle back toward my car.

"Hey!" he calls out. "Are you *okay*?"

There's no telling how long he had been watching me, but his eyes tell me that he is not going to let me get in my car and drive away until he gets a satisfactory answer. My brain is too tired to generate a believable lie, so I tell the truth.

"I know Amanda from church and I need to talk to her. I tried knocking, but nobody answered and I don't want to ring the doorbell and wake up the kids."

"Do you want me to call her?" he asks.

"I don't have their phone number." My arms shrug.

"I have it." He disappears into his house.

Remarkable. I don't have any of my neighbors' phone numbers.

My legs have made a dozen pivots, like an army private practicing about-face, trying to decide if it's not too late to back out of the whole thing, when he returns.

"Derek answered. He's coming down to open the door."

"Thank you." I mean it.

Deadbolts unlock on the other side and a wedge of space opens, revealing half of Derek's face, nose and one eye, searching to identify the form standing on his doorstep at this hour.

"Hi," I say weakly. "I'm sorry to wake you so late, I tried to knock quietly, but no one answered and the neighbor saw me and offered to call you." The words rush out, running together, and I'm trying not to let my voice crack. "Is Amanda awake?"

The door opens wider. "Come in." Amanda yawns behind Derek. She is the brightest, most bubbly, most energetic person I've ever met, and I somehow expected she would even be bright and energetic in her sleep. Coming was a bad idea.

"Come in," she says again.

She moves pillows and pats a seat for me on her couch before she finally appears to realize who I am. "Maleah! What's up?"

"Is there anything I can do?" Derek asks, wondering his place in all of this.

"Would you call Aaron and tell him I'm here?" At the mention of Aaron's name, Derek places my face. He dials as I recite the cell number. I listen while Derek has a conversation with my husband about me while I'm sitting in the room.

"He says he's glad you're here." Derek gives Amanda a look before going upstairs, and I have the impression they've danced this routine before. Is it possible I'm not the only woman who has turned up in pajamas and tennis shoes on their doorstep after midnight?

"Maleah, did you just have a baby?" Amanda asks, and I realize again how long it's been since we've talked to each other. So why did I think of coming here? "What's going on?" she prompts.

"I…" What are the words?

"Do you have postpartum depression?"

The question doesn't sound accusatory coming from her. "I don't know. I don't think so. I don't feel depressed. Mostly I'm tired. My doctor asked if I wanted Wellbutrin, but my family has strange reactions to medication. I'm afraid a drug will make me worse."

She once announced to the whole Sunday School class that she and Derek kiss her Prozac bottle every morning. At the time I felt embarrassed for her, but she related the fact as if she were confessing that she dislikes broccoli or has overdue library books.

We talk a long while. If Amanda is eager to get back to bed, she doesn't let on.

"I don't want happiness from a bottle. I don't want life from a bottle. I want the real thing, not an artificial substitute."

"The medicine doesn't make me feel fake, it allows me to be the real me."

I nod. Amanda is the polar opposite of fake. "I don't want to be dependent on a drug."

"If you were diabetic, would you refuse insulin?" she asks.

The more we talk, the better I feel. The threat of explosion has been diffused. The drumming in my chest has softened to a regular rhythm. Breath flows past my throat without constriction. "Thank you. I'd better let you get back to bed." I stand to leave.

"Promise you'll make an appointment to see your doctor and then call me." Amanda gives me a hug. "That doesn't mean you have to take medicine, but go find out more."

I promise.

Before getting in my car I look at the fence. No one is there. "Thank you," I say to the space where the head had been earlier. I don't know who he is or why he was looking over his fence at that hour, but he saved my life.

On the drive home, I marvel how therapeutic it felt sitting on Amanda's couch, putting words to the dust storm in my brain. She didn't make me feel crazy. She made my neurosis feel normal. The agitation, the ticking bomb is gone. A peaceful exhaustion settles over me.

At home Aaron is in bed, but he's not asleep.

"You okay?" he asks.

"Yeah." I take a breath to be sure. "I feel better."

IN THE MORNING Laiah asks if I'm worried that Amanda is on the phone with someone from church, gossiping away about the crazy visit she had last night. "What if she uses you as an example in a Sunday School lesson?" Laiah speaks as if word getting out would be more of an embarrassment to her than to me. Amanda won't tell a soul. At this moment I picture her kissing the garbage can mark on Derek's forehead before he leaves for work and this image makes me feel hopeful. Amanda has been where I am, and she came out okay on the other side.

In fact, this morning I feel so much better—no crawling skin, no blood ready to boil, no mental tornado—that calling Dr. Woods' office seems absurd, but Amanda made me promise. My message on the answering machine has barely disconnected when the phone rings in my hand with the nurse practitioner returning my call. She talks to me for a long time and won't let me hang up until she knows I won't harm myself or Jack and have agreed to come into the office. At the appointment she, like Dr. Woods, offers a prescription for Wellbutrin. I'm nervous about medication, I tell her, and want to wait and see if things improve on their own.

Laiah says that hard work is the best way to cure depression, so if I keep working hard and this goes away, then I'll know it was depression. If I work hard and this *doesn't* go away, then I'll know there must be something more seriously wrong with me than depression. This is my plan as Aaron and I work our way through the November and December issues of the magazine.

CHAPTER 28

Emergency Surgery

THE GREMLINS OF the universe have discovered that print deadline is the third weekend of every month, and those imps have figured out how to manipulate time so that any crisis coming our way falls exactly on that weekend. On the third Friday in November, a car pulls in front of our house and delivers Danny from his after-school play date. Danny slams the front door and drops his backpack in the middle of the kitchen floor where it lands with a *thud*.

"Danny, what have you got in there?"

He unzips his pack and one at a time removes every book from the thirty-two-volume *Magic Tree House* set, one of the presents for his seventh birthday last month. Danny lifts the stack, but flinches in pain. "Mom, when I cough or sneeze my stomach hurts right here." He pats his lower stomach.

"Did you fall or get hit anywhere today?"

"When I jumped down from the monkey bars it hurt really bad."

"Let me take a look." Aaron kneels and Danny lowers his shorts. His groin is swollen to the size of a small cantaloupe. Aaron and I look at each other. It's after 5:00; our pediatrician's office is closed for the weekend. "I'll take him to the emergency room at Del Webb," Aaron offers.

"No! Not Del Webb. I've heard too many horror stories lately about the ER there." At church Crystal had recounted the nightmare of taking her son to the Del Webb emergency room over the weekend.

He was unconscious and burning up and they still waited five hours. Rachel, my piano student/newspaper reporter told me about a man who died in line waiting to be seen. "Drive him to Phoenix Children's. It will take an hour to get there, but you'll see a doctor faster."

When Aaron carries Danny through the automatic doors at Phoenix Children's Hospital, the staff wastes no time ushering him in for tests. Aaron calls from the triage room. Danny has a testicular torsion. He is scheduled for immediate surgery. Making an uncommon exception to standard procedure, a surgeon arrives at the hospital to perform the midnight operation. A few more hours and they wouldn't have been able to save the teste. Interesting how for appendicitis, heart trauma, or any other organ, the patient would have waited out the night for a surgeon's daytime working hours, but not in this case. When it comes to saving man parts, those surgeons take the area pretty seriously.

The next morning Aaron reports that Danny is out of bed and happily exploring the playroom. If his vitals are good, they'll release him this afternoon.

"Thank you for being there with him," I tell Aaron. Today was supposed to be Aaron's time to lay-out the December magazine.

There's no choice but to pack Kate, Tanner, and Jack into the van and drag them along to my last-minute business visits. They wait in the car with the air conditioner running while I gather approval signatures on final ad proofs.

"Mom, I'm bored," Kate moans after the third stop.

"Guys, I know. You're being so patient."

Danny arrives home with an armful of new stuffed animals and gift bags of goodies giving us the impression he's coming home from an amusement park rather than a hospital. We are updated on all the fabulous amenities offered at PCH including a study table in the game room where you could do schoolwork—which he did, even though it was Saturday and he didn't miss any school. "You should go there," Danny tells Kate. She can hardly wait.

Aaron has nothing but good to say about the experience. "Everybody was amazing. They got us right in and knew exactly what they were doing. I'm so glad you said to go there. If I'd taken him to Del Webb and waited for hours, we might have a fifty percent less chance of being grandparents."

Aaron's positive report causes me to think about Kate's tonsillectomy. Maybe the insurance glitch happened for a reason. There have been so many stories lately of botched procedures on kids at Del Webb Hospital, and who's to say it's their fault? In Sun City West they're equipped to deal with heart attacks, kidney failure, and diabetes. Phoenix Children's specializes in kids. Their surgical tables and equipment are sized for kids. Does Del Webb have smaller surgical instruments, or do they force adult-sized scalpels down children's throats? Maybe Danny's surgery is a sign to find a different doctor for Kate, one who does tonsillectomies at Phoenix Children's instead of Del Webb.

Aaron stays awake all night Sunday finishing the Christmas issue. In the morning I meet him in the office where he hands me the printed stack of pages to proofread. "I'm going to sleep for a few hours. Wake me up when you're done proofing and I'll upload it to the printers."

Danny wakes on his own and is dressed and ready fifteen minutes early. He can hardly wait to share the details of his emergency hospital visit for first grade show and tell. If I were a responsible mother, I might escort him to class and warn his teacher, but I'm pushed up against a deadline. What will Mrs. Gordon do when Danny walks to the front and tells his classmates the story of his engorged testicle?

—◦◦◦—

THE STAGE GLOWS inside a halo of white holiday lights and garland. From the ninth row, my eyes scan the room assessing the decorations for tonight's piano recital. Laiah holds her thumb in front of her nose taking a visual measurement between the two poinsettia plants, making sure they are an equal distance from the microphone. The piano lid is raised, the doughnuts and hot chocolate are set to serve, but I am not at all ready for this, my final piano recital. I collapse into the seat, my head bonking on the back of the wooden bench.

All day my body has struggled to move. Last night I thought the body aches were from stress combined with the sadness of abandoning my students. The weekend of Danny's surgery threw me behind schedule and I haven't been able to catch up since. His emergency is what ultimately led me to decide to stop teaching piano lessons. Our life has no wiggle room for unexpected incidents—and with kids there are always unexpected incidents. Finally coming to terms with what I'd been denying for too long, my piano students received—in the same envelope—an invitation to the Christmas recital as well as an official note announcing December as my last month of teaching. The phone calls followed. Mrs. Vanderhost begged me to please keep Brianna. "She's never found anything she loves so much as piano. She has completely changed. She's confident. Her grades are straight A's now." I hung up the phone, slid down the cabinet into the pile of napkins Jack had pulled from the dispenser, folded my head over my knees, and wished for the kind of good cry that would make me feel better. But I hadn't been able to cry.

Laiah reminded me that most women are achy and tired while breastfeeding. "It's normal," she said, but this morning my throat felt like I'd swallowed a belt sander and left it running all night. On the way to pick up recital refreshments, I stopped into the newly opened urgent care swearing that if the doctor asked me one thing about a newborn or slightly hinted at the word *antidepressant*, I might burn the building down. Certainly a sore throat could not be mistaken for postpartum depression.

The physician probed my neck and shined her spotlight onto the dark recesses in the back of my throat. "Your glands are swollen.

By the looks of things back there I'm ninety-nine percent certain you have strep throat, but our lab technician is gone for an extended weekend, so I could make you wait and come back Monday for the throat swab and culture to be one hundred percent certain, or I could give you a prescription now, and you'll be better by Monday."

"Give me the drugs, *please*," I'd said. Taking an anti*biotic* was nothing like taking an anti*depressant*. She handed me the script with a caution that I'd be contagious for twenty-four hours after swallowing the first pill.

Here I am, six hours later, greeting parents and students, shaking hands and passing out programs, trying not to breathe germs when I hug them and say, "Merry Christmas," which is a challenge since this is the last time I will see many of them.

CHAPTER 29

Minivan Caravan

WE CELEBRATE AN early Christmas at home on December 19, which is also Day of the Deadline, a time when Aaron and I walk around like the living dead. The sun is barely up when the kids jump onto our bed shouting about presents in the living room. "Santa left a note!" Danny shoves a paper into my face, but I already know what it says. Using my best Santa penmanship, I had written: *Dear Warners, Thought you might not have room in your van to bring everything home from Utah, so I delivered a few gifts early. Santa.*

An hour later the family room looks like a shaken snow globe: Flurries of wrapping paper, ribbons, bows, and packaging float through the air among squeals of excitement. While the kids play, Aaron disappears into the office and returns with the rough draft of our January issue. "Good luck proofreading. Let me know when you finish." Wearing shorts and a T-shirt, he goes outside to get the yardwork done before we leave town. The kids, also wearing shorts and tees, take their new Christmas toys outside to play on the sunny patio.

Two days and a ten-hour drive later, we are bundled nose to toes in snow gear and are tubing down Aaron's favorite childhood sledding hill. I didn't want to travel to Utah for Christmas this year. The strep throat on top of everything else made staying home tucked in my bed seem like the greatest Christmas gift in the world. But all month I crossed off squares of the December calendar waiting for the opportune moment to speak the rehearsed words: "Aaron, let's have Christmas at home," which I finally mustered the courage to speak at midnight on December 19, *while* packing our suitcases. By then the wheels were already in motion and it was too late to stop the trip. The only thing my words accomplished was creating a tense ten-hour drive.

And here's the very reason I didn't want to travel to Utah:

On December 26, I'm hauling the last suitcase up the stairs of my in-laws' house when I hear Aaron answer his cell phone. "We're leaving in about an hour," he speaks into his phone. "Sure, that would be great. Where do you want to meet up? Sure thing. See you then. Bye." He puts the phone in his pocket. "That was your mom. They are getting ready to leave and wondered if we want to caravan."

"They aren't leaving until tomorrow." I prop the suitcase against the wall and go to the bottom of the stairs for the duffle bag.

"Your brother got extra time off work, so everybody wants to leave a day earlier."

The entire Day family clan—the whole fam damily, as the expression goes—is coming to spend New Year's in Arizona. There will be somewhere around thirty-six people (each time I count, I come up with a different number) and Annice and I are housing and feeding them *all*.

The duffel bag on my shoulder bangs the stair railing as I pound up the stairs. "We have to leave NOW!" I shout. "Put this in the car. Grab the kids." Aaron steps back when the duffle hits his chest.

I send the kids through a hasty assembly line of goodbye hugs and kisses and leave my in-laws with their mouths gaping at our speedy departure. Aaron is confused, but I absolutely must get to my house before company arrives. There's no milk in the fridge. The mantle will be dusty. Aaron also lives in the house, but when company comes, anything dirty, moldy, smelly, or out-of-stock is a reflection on me.

"Come on, come on." My leg bounces as I hold open the front door waving for Aaron, who loiters, talking with his dad. I'm a cowgirl digging spurs into her horse's flanks—my horse may be a 2001 Ford Minivan, but still, the bandits are hot on my tail.

Once we're cruising in a rhythm on the freeway and Jack has fallen asleep, I shift my weight in the seat and lean my head back, which loosens a mass of sinus drainage and triggers another coughing fit. Usually antibiotics work like a charm for me and in two days I feel so much better that it's hard to take the full ten-day prescription, though I always do. This time I've finished the ten days of antibiotics but don't feel any better from the strep throat.

As we approach Las Vegas, Aaron's phone rings. It's my brother, Karl. They've caught up to us. "They want to meet up for lunch," Aaron whispers to me. I shake my head, but hear Aaron say, "We'll meet you at the Burger King off the exit." I glare at Aaron. "The kids have to eat." He shrugs.

The cousins ignore their fries in favor of chasing each other around the play land. My stomach churns nauseous thinking about the amount of snot and germs that have been wiped inside those slides. So help me if extended family spends the week battling stomach flu in my bathrooms. After eating, the cousins trade vehicles according to age groups for the duration of the trip. Our parade of minivans snakes around the Grand Canyon looking like a circus train brimming with luggage and the hands and feet of wild monkeys waving wildly out the window.

We make it to Wickenburg, Arizona, before the kids start fighting about who gets to use the bathroom first when we get home. Jack wakes up crying. "Should we stop so you can feed him?" Aaron asks. "We could tell your family where to find the spare house key."

No! I have to get to my house before my company does. I need to make sure bank account statements are hidden away and that our preferred method of family planning is not sitting on the bathroom counter. "No stopping. Drive faster." Rummaging through the diaper bag I find stray Cheerios and pieces of broken graham cracker to appease Jack. By the time we turn off Grand Avenue my nerves are beyond frazzled. Aaron is hunched over the steering wheel, his knuckles white. The most appealing thing in the world would be to take a steamy shower and clear up my clogged sinuses, soothe my aching muscles, then slide on pajamas and bury myself under my own bed covers.

What am I going to feed all these people for dinner?

THE CONVOY OF vehicles converges around our house like a SWAT team. Kids fall out of car doors (invoking images of clowns spilling out from Volkswagens) and begin doing a cross-legged jumping routine. What must look like a bizarre tribal ritual to the neighbors peering discretely through cracks in blinds is actually a potty dance. "Dad, hurry!" the kids shout, squeezing their legs tighter. The key to the front door falls from my hand. Jack, in his car seat, is deposited on the kitchen tile while I wash and disinfect my hands. His little face is red with hunger and anger, his droopy diaper makes him weigh twice as much as usual, but he'll never make it through a diaper change. Food first.

Settling into breastfeeding basecamp, I whisper "Shh, shh," in his ear adjusting my shirt so he can latch on before he hyperventilates. There is noise in the kitchen—*my terrain!*—and my head shoots up, nose sniffs the air, shoulders raise, neck hairs stand alert. The refrigerator is open. I'm a territorial dog tracking a trespasser.

"Mom, I'm hungry. What's for dinner?"

"Close the fridge!" I order. "Go clean out the van."

The kids scatter to the playroom and dump out the toy buckets.

The sound of the fridge opening again alerts my ears.

"CLOSE THAT FRIDGE!" I yell.

My sister-in-law, Caroline, turns to me sheepishly and closes the fridge.

"I'm sorry. I thought you were the kids. What do you need?" My tone of voice changes, but my claws have come out like switchblades.

"Maleah, do you have any milk?"

What I *want* to say is this: "Yes, I have milk, but it's being used at the moment. Can you wait your turn?"

Instead, I say pointedly—to remind everyone that I have not been home for a week. "We got rid of the milk before we left for Christmas, didn't want sour milk. (Duh!) Let me finish feeding Jack and I'll go to the store."

Laiah breezes in looking refreshed and perfect, not travel-weary at all. She sits on the arm of the couch. "What's stopping Caroline from going to the store? She has two arms and a driver's license."

Meanwhile my bladder is rolling like a water balloon threatening to burst and I consider carrying Jack to the bathroom and relieving myself while he eats, but judging by the continual toilet flushes, the lineup for my two bathrooms is wrapping down the hallway.

Caroline fills her toddler's sippy cup with ice water instead of milk. The ice and water dispenser on my fridge has been grinding non-stop since we came in. The sink is piling up with used cups, my guests falsely assuming that I have enough drinking glasses for them to luxuriously dirty one now, toss it in the sink, and get a new, clean glass for dinner.

Next, it's Aaron who pulls the fridge door open assessing the depravity of our grocery situation. My fridge is being ransacked while I'm trapped in breastfeeding confinement. "I'll run and grab milk," Aaron says. "What else do we need from the store?"

My nerves spike like quills on a porcupine. Why won't everyone just chill and wait fifteen minutes? I wish for the superpower to freeze everybody where they are so I can finish breastfeeding in peace.

"What we *need* is for everybody to go away," Laiah gripes under her breath.

There are so many things we need from the store, probably a two-hour shopping trip with multiple carts filled to the brim, but at this moment, other than milk, I can't think of a single item. I reach back into my brain and try to access the mental shopping list I'd made before leaving town, but my brain is too fragmented. Pieces of my cerebral cortex are still in Christmas, some got stuck in the printer jam with my piano recital program, other bits are hanging out at the mailing office with our January magazine, and I'm sure there are remnants I never brought home from the hospital after Jack was born.

"Aaron, can't you wait a bit?" I need a minute of solitude to gather my brain cells or at least muster the few remaining troops. "No one is going to die of starvation in the next five minutes."

"I'll just go get milk and you can do the rest of the shopping later." Aaron grabs the other set of car keys and charges out the front door.

"No!" I shout, but I'm not sure if I scream out loud or in my head. I don't want to do the rest of the shopping later, but he's already gone, headed for the peace and tranquility of the grocery store, leaving me alone in this den of starving lions.

"Maleah, where do you want this?" My good-hearted nephew lumbers in under the weight of two large suitcases. He is singlehandedly unloading my van.

A call comes from down the hall. "Maleah, where do you keep more toilet paper?"

Toilet paper! I'd forgotten to buy toilet paper.

"Aaron!" I yell—out loud for sure this time. The shout startles Jack, who comes unlatched and pauses briefly, scrunching up his face before breaking into the full howl we'd listened to for the last hour of the car ride. "Benji!" I call to my nephew. "Go see if Uncle Aaron drove away yet. If not, tell him we need toilet paper."

Benji calls from the front door, "He already left."

Jack's powerful cries loosen something in his belly. He grunts and bears down. Three days of constipation—this is going to be a doozy.

"Aunt Maleah." My niece enters holding a box of mutilated crayons in her pinched fingers like she's found a dead animal. "Tanner had this in his mouth." The box is ripped and soggy, punctured into the shape of a toddler dental imprint. Tanner runs into the room and bares his teeth, revealing a rainbow Crayola grin; the tips of several new crayons are wedged between his canines. "And he smells bad," she complains.

Poor Tanner. He hasn't had his diaper changed since our Vegas break almost six hours ago.

"That's embarrassing," Laiah quips. "Now all your sisters-in-law will know that Tanner isn't potty trained yet. He's two and a half."

A glance at the microwave clock tells me it's almost 7:30 p.m. We'd been on the road for over twelve hours when we usually made it in under ten. My parents drive the speed limit. Without caravanning I could have gotten home two hours ago and grocery shopped already.

"Watch out!" a panicked voice calls from the garage. An enormous crash is followed by the ricochet of spilling toys. The taller cousins have reached up to the highest shelf and dumped out the bin of toys that I'd spent weeks sorting and cleaning to donate to Goodwill. Now they will be mixed with the other toys and made dirty again.

The decibel level in my house thunders louder than a rock concert, but it's not louder than the rumble which pulls my attention back to the infant in my lap. In the nick of time I pull Jack away from my breast and hold him over a blanket as a three-day sewage backup erupts and brown goop oozes out of his pants. Heading for my bedroom and the changing table, I am holding Jack like hazardous waste at arms' length in front of me when my sister-in-law passes me in the hallway.

"Maleah, just tell me what you want me to do for dinner and I'll do it."

"What do you want me to do. What do you want me to do," Laiah mimics her like a parrot, then turns to me. "Remember that talk we had about planning ahead. Here is the perfect example of how you could be better organized. People were expecting you to be more prepared, especially Aaron. Ooooh"—she shivers as if a chill crawled up her spine just thinking about it—"you could sense how stressed out and disappointed he was when he left for the store."

Right there in the hallway, I share with Laiah a joyful hallucination in which I pick up the phone and order a dozen pizzas—enough different types of pizza that every niece, nephew, cousin, brother, sister-in-law, parent (and any homeless person who might wander in unnoticed) will shut up and eat. Laiah interrupts my delivery daydream to remind me of my place in the too-poor-to-order-pizza club. Our bank account is already behind from Christmas. Quitting piano means no lesson income for January, and I haven't yet accrued enough ad revenue to replace Aaron's Cloverman income. I don't have enough money to buy pizza for this crowd.

Laiah tries to be helpful. "Quit whining. You can brainstorm something cheap and simple to make for dinner, but it should be moderately fancy, these are your guests." Laiah is not dishing out anything I haven't asked her to lay on me. I have to figure out how to quit letting people down.

My sister-in-law shadows me into my bedroom where I lay an old towel over the changing table and peel Jack like a spoiled banana. "Um, what sounds good for dinner?" I say, faking nonchalance. "We've been snacking so much on the drive I don't feel very hungry." In truth, I am ravenous and imagine Aaron with barbecue tongs pulling a thick steak off the grill, which I grab with bare hands and devour on the spot then reach out for a second.

In the end we eat plain spaghetti (no meatballs) and green beans from a can—all stuff from the pantry. After dinner I spend an hour wiping marinara sauce off the walls, chairs, carpet, and couch.

—◦◦◦—

ON THE LAST night with our houseguests, I use the stockpile of coupons the owner of China Gourmet has been giving me to pay for her ad. One phone call and the restaurant delivers rice for a battalion.

My mother offers a blessing on the food and I pray in my heart that Aaron will miraculously find something among the multiple trays of Chinese food that he'll want to eat. As people fill their plates, I run sprints between the garage and the kitchen, grabbing ranch dressing, ketchup, bread with butter and jam—all the Day family essentials that don't come standard with an international meal.

At last I land in a corner seat with what remained of the sweet and sour pork. On the other side of the garage Aaron mashes a plastic spoon into his untasted food. He seems like a stranger to me. We've hardly spoken in days. Annice carries her half-finished plate toward me. "You're over here by yourself." She pulls out the metal folding chair next to me. These past five days our only conversations have been about who was going to sleep, eat, shower, and be entertained where, when, and how.

"The kids' table is my level tonight," I try to make a joke.

"Are you okay, Maleah?" Annice asks. She isn't making light table talk; she is asking sincerely.

"I'm just…" What are the words? There's no description for what is wrong with me. My feet move, my arms work, but I'm dragging my body like Linus drags his blue blanket. This is something I've never experienced before. I'm tired in a way I've never been tired before. My bone marrow is tired. The best answer I come up with to Annice's question is, "I am just…so…tired."

LAST NOVEMBER OUR friends Marsha and Keith hosted all of their extended family for Thanksgiving. When Marsha surfaced several days later, I asked how the weekend had gone. She told me in a still-weary voice that they had used every linen in the house: every sheet, pillowcase, hand towel, dish rag, washcloth. "We did not have a crumb of bread or a drop of milk left. For three days I did nothing but get things for people. When they left, Keith and I went to bed and slept for two days."

My parents are the last to leave. My dad bends down for his hug. "I hope I have your mom convinced that we should buy a house and move down here during the winter. My back can't handle shoveling snow like it used to." We wave until their car disappears around the corner.

Back in the house I stare at the empty rooms. My family has gone, taking their piles of luggage and their comforting distraction. *What now?* I fantasize about crawling back into bed, wrapping myself around a pillow, and sinking into deep sleep. Laiah emerges from the hall holding two hangers of possible business outfits. Part of our *Get Maleah Organized* plan is to choose wardrobe in advance so I don't waist precious minutes—my rarest commodity—stuck in the closet, hemming and hawing over what to wear. Today I have to get tear sheets delivered. Per Bob's praxis, each month we hand-carry to each customer a copy of the newest issue with a tear-out page showing their ad, along with an invoice.

"Green slacks or purple skirt." Laiah alternately holds out the options.

Kate taps my leg. "Mom, play a game?" She holds a deck of Old Maid cards. Behind her Tanner waits, eyes lit with excitement, eager to be included in the game, hopeful to be dealt a hand including his favorite card, *Postman Pete.* The kids have one more week of school break. They have been entertained and distracted for fourteen days, smothered with attention and drowning in play.

"Mommy has so much to do today."

Kate's chin drops to her chest; the sparkle falls from her face.

CHAPTER 30

I Need a Mother

OVER THE PAST five months, I've spent every Friday morning eating greasy eggs and burnt hash browns at a country diner, mingling with other business members of the Southwest Valley Chamber of Commerce. After months on the waitlist, today is finally my turn to do the breakfast business spotlight. The presentation I've worked up will hopefully be attention-grabbing, interactive, and memorable. I want every person in that room holding one of my magazines in their hot little hands, flipping through the pages, reading the content, and seeing their competitors' beautiful full-page ad on the inside front cover. They might think they are only playing a fast-paced search-and-find game in order to win a chocolate bar, but in reality they will be falling in love with the newest monthly in town.

On the way to school, flashing lights signal for me to pull over. I turn into the school parking lot and let Danny and Kate run into class so they don't have to witness my interlude with the law. The policeman walks to my car in slow motion. *Come on Officer, let's make this a fast conversation about speeding because I have a million things to do today.* After a lecture and verbal warning, the officer follows behind as I drive carefully out of the lot. The minute his patrol car turns the opposite direction, the gas pedal meets the floor.

Pulling in front of the diner, I wonder if I can set up in time for my presentation. My arms, usually capable of lifting fifty-pound bags of flour without problem, strain to heft the box with one hundred copies of our January issue. Making several trips from the restaurant to the trunk, I carry in business cards, rate sheets, advertising contracts, a game buzzer, and prizes.

The buffet is surrounded by business owners who are older and more experienced in business than I am. Being pulled over has left me nervous and unsettled. In the bathroom I stuff paper towels under my arms so my blouse won't show sweat marks. My neck is breaking out in red, nervous blotches. I fluff my hair, wipe smeared mascara from beneath my eyes, freshen lipstick, and take deep breaths. *Stop shaking.*

The chamber president introduces me.

"Hi friends." My legs wobble. "Is everyone ready to play an awesome game this morning?"

Following the presentation, I sell three new ads and the mayor asks me to be on the committee to plan the upcoming chamber trade show. The crowd around me lingers. Despite my best efforts to appear calm and in control, I have broken out in chills, my teeth won't stop chattering, the paper towels under my arms are drenched. "I'd better get going," I say at last.

Phillipe, an odd man who introduces a new business enterprise every few weeks, stands when I do. "Let me take one of those boxes for you." He follows me making small talk then asks unexpectedly, "Are you still married?"

My shoe catches on a crack in the pavement, the tower in my arms leans, and I weave right and left to counterbalance. Phillipe waits for my answer. "Um…yes, I am still married. Why do you ask?"

"I noticed you aren't wearing your wedding ring anymore," he says, pointing to my left hand.

"Oh. That." The photo frames tip over in the box. "I've lost some weight and my ring keeps sliding off. I don't want to lose it."

Phillipe proceeds to tell me about a jeweler he's partnering with who adjusts ring sizes. He puts the box in the trunk and hands me a business card, which I plan to throw away. No reason to resize my ring because once I stop nursing Jack, the weight will come right back.

The heat in my car is blasting full power, but I can't stop shivering. It's almost noon, later than I told Aaron I would be. Dizzy and disoriented, I make two wrong turns before getting onto the main road. The gas empty light flashes angrily, but Jack is going to be starving. No time to refuel.

WHEN I TURN the corner onto Memory Lane, Aaron is in the front yard pacing the length of the grass and bouncing Jack. Tanner scoots a sit-on fire engine up and down the sidewalk. Jack's face is red, his cheeks soggy with tears. I rush to them, lifting Jack from Aaron's shoulder. "Hey there. Shhh. It's okay." I kiss his face. "Did you try giving him a binky?" I question Aaron.

"You know he won't take a binky. There's nothing I can do for him when he's hungry. If you think you'll be late, you've got to leave me a bottle."

I had tried to pump that morning, but didn't have extra milk. "I didn't know I would be so long. People stayed after breakfast to ask about advertising. I have three new ads for you to design."

Aaron picks up Tanner's fire engine and we enter through the garage. I'm unbuttoning my blouse and Jack is trying to latch on as we walk.

"Maybe it's time to stop nursing." Aaron bites a loose piece of dry skin on his lower lip.

His comment at once disarms me and sets off my defenses. "Breast milk is healthiest for Jack. Buying formula would cost fifty dollars a month."

"But you don't have enough milk for him."

With all my strength I hold in tears so Aaron won't see me cry. I fire back, "That's because we went to Utah for Christmas. Traveling always makes me lose my milk." The last thing I want to consider is the possibility that Aaron might be right. I've failed at so many things, I can't fail in breastfeeding as well. Caught off-guard and unable to govern my emotions, I make the mistake of telling Aaron about the dizziness in the parking lot as I carry Jack to the bedroom.

"Why won't you go to a doctor?" Aaron's question follows me down the hall where I take Jack and settle into my bedroom rocking chair without answering.

In the rocker Jack sucks furiously, but there is no milk. In all the dashing here and there this morning, my milk hasn't let down. Jack unlatches, looks at me questioningly, and resumes crying. I squeeze my nipple to coax milk to come, but instead of creamy white liquid sustenance, only clear, fat tears land on Jack's mouth. His tongue flicks out to lick the drops, then he squints and recoils at the salty taste.

Why won't I go to a doctor?

A KNOCK AT my bedroom door gets my attention and Laiah comes to sit by me during this feeble attempt at nursing. "Aaron asked why I won't I go to a doctor," I tell her. "How does a person know if they're sick *enough* to merit seeing a doctor?"

That was the standard go-to question my siblings and I could expect to hear our mom ask if we mentioned staying home from school. "Do you think you're sick enough to miss school?" I never knew how to answer. What was the measure of sick *enough*? My family rolled our eyes while using the term "hypochondriac" to describe people who went to the doctor for every fever or sniffle. There were days working in the field when I watched my dad bent over an irrigation ditch puking so violently I expected to see him barf up a kidney. Secretly I hoped he would call it a day so I could go inside and watch cartoons, but before the echo of his retching had finished bouncing off the castle valley hills, he had wiped his mouth on his shirt sleeve, replaced his work hat, and was asking why I hadn't yet fetched him the wire cutters.

Growing up, even being legitimately sick didn't necessarily justify seeing a doctor, or missing work or school. Every July on Pioneer Day we venerated our ancestors who pushed handcarts through blizzards with frostbitten hands and feet long past the time their human strength had given out. No matter how deep I sift through my files of recollection, I cannot find one memory of either my mom or dad spending a day in bed for being sick. But I can easily pull up one of the worst memories from my ninth-grade year—an image and a deep, bellowing voice that still make me cringe in disgrace.

That morning I'd woken with a fever and sore throat. Mom asked if I felt sick *enough* to stay home from school. The answer was yes, but there was too much happening at school to miss—an algebra test, a history report, and an after-school dance team practice. By lunch my head was throbbing so hard that instead of going to wood shop class, I went to the office and asked to lie down. The secretary said she'd call my mom to come get me. No, I said, I needed to stay at school and take my test, but if I could just rest for forty-five minutes. The nurse escorted me back to a couch and offered medicine. I declined the medicine, accepted the couch, and fell asleep, to be awakened by the booming bass voice of the assistant principal.

"Which faker do we have in here today?" The question was directed to the secretary regarding the sleeping form on the couch, the words ringing like low tones from a bell tower. To this day, when I hear the voice of actor James Earl Jones, I feel a shiver of guilt run up my spine remembering the dagger of accusation. "Who is the lazy bones faking sick and sluffing class?"

There could be no lower esteem of my character than to be thought a lazy faker. I sat up from the couch—my head reeling—went to class, answered foggy algebra test questions, and somehow spun my way through drill team rehearsal.

The next day Mom took me to the one and only clinic in town. I don't remember the diagnosis, I only remember the feeling of utter relief when the town doctor declared, "This is one sick girl." The school received a doctor's note—written evidence against the allegation of faking and laziness.

But what if the doctor hadn't found anything wrong with me?

I try to shake the memory and relax so that my milk will let down, but my breasts are limp and empty. Jack's face wrinkles into a cry. "Aaron is right. I should stop nursing. He needs a bottle of formula."

"Hang in there," Laiah urges. "You've wanted for a long time to nurse a baby the full twelve months. This is just a setback. Give Jack formula today and you'll lose your milk for good. Keep trying. His rooting will stimulate lactation."

She is also right. My mother breastfed eight babies. When she calls, no matter what else we discuss, she always asks if I'm still nursing. Motherhood is not about doing what feels good. Motherhood is synonymous with sacrifice.

THE REST OF the day is rough, and I don't sleep well that night. Saturday morning Aaron leaps out of bed. In no time the lawn mower is passing back and forth outside my bedroom window. He didn't look at me, feel my forehead, test to see if I was breathing, ask if I'm okay this morning after a rough night. This fact that he didn't check on me rubs at a tender interior part until I sting raw like skinned knuckles after getting too close to a cheese grater.

Laiah enters with her hair freshly washed, rubbing lotion into her arms. I tell her about the cold absence of a simple good morning. "Aaron resents me. I annoy him."

"Maybe he's letting you sleep in." Laiah tries to find the bright side.

If he thought I was sleeping, then he is clueless about how little I sleep. Laiah isn't clueless. She knows how I spend hours in the night, hovering above the surface of sleep, like floating above a warm feather duvet and being close enough to sense its pillowy softness, but unable to be engulfed in its layers of comfort.

"He doesn't love me anymore."

"He has a lot to do today."

"So his backyard deserves more attention than his wife?" In the other room Danny and Tanner are awake jumping on their beds. How can I get a portion of their energy?

"I suppose if he believed you were sick then he wouldn't have abandoned you in the house with the natives." Laiah nods toward Danny's bedroom, where the sound of the mattress sliding off its box springs makes me realize that mowing a lawn would require a lot less effort than wrestling the kids through their morning routine. At least Laiah can now see the proof. Aaron wasn't making a kind gesture by letting me sleep in, he has locked himself in the quiet outdoors, leaving me here alone to handle the herd.

"He doesn't believe I'm sick?" Aaron didn't offer to take the kids this morning so I could sleep because he doesn't believe me; he doesn't think it's real when I try to describe how awful I feel. "Does he think I'm *faking*?" My face darkens. Aaron is ignoring me on purpose.

When I stand, a searing headache shoots across my scalp. Swallowing is a million needles hammered into my esophagus. A fit of coughing sends me running for the toilet to relieve my bladder before the coughing does it for me. The coughing loosens layers of phlegm that leaves me leaning over my bathroom sink, spitting and wiping mucus from my chin. In the mirror the eyes of a wild Amazon woman with pale, acne-marked skin gaze at me. *Look at me now, Aaron. Bet you can't photoshop this.* No wonder Aaron prefers spending time with the greener grass on the outside of our little white house than being cooped up in here with his wilting wife. Who could blame him for wanting to be in a place with a little more life?

The room spins. Jack fusses. Tanner and Danny launch into my room like bottle rockets and bounce on the bed. My arms buckle lifting Jack out of the crib and I have to immediately lay him on the floor not to drop him. This sets him to crying harder. Danny leaps from the bed, taking me down in a sneak tackle from behind. The sounds of needy voices echo off the walls calling for food, drink, attention, dry diapers, but I have nothing to give. My throat goes sour with resentment for Aaron leaving me in the house alone. The lawn can go to hell—he should be in here working crowd control.

Danny's tackle has left me splayed out in the middle of my bedroom floor in a loose fetal position with legs spread askew. My arm reaches out and pulls Jack to my chest. He wiggles and roots until he finds one breast and sucks vigorously for several minutes until, in frustration, he lets go and looks up at me, his bottom lip quivering. I blow lightly on his hair. Tears roll down my temple and moisten my arm before melting into the carpet. Jack is crying. We are hungry, but neither of us knows what to do about it.

I may not be green and lush, but I need Aaron more than I need a green lawn. I need someone to lift me up, wrap me in a blanket, hold me safe in their arms, rocking and soothing me, whispering that everything will be okay.

I need a mother.

Book Three

Change

CHAPTER 31

Ears to Hear

THE LAST WEEK of January, Kate holds my hand nervously as we walk into the office of a new ear, nose, and throat specialist. Following instructions, she climbs up into a large leather chair and sits bravely answering questions with a smile, ever eager to please. She doesn't fill half the chair, but the exam room overflows with her energy and light. Her entrance into any space conjures images of sunshine rays shooting through a prism and ricocheting as vibrant rainbows off multiple surfaces at once. My lips whisper a silent prayer that this doctor will be able to help Kate. She is radiance and love despite the constant dark circles under her eyes and her tonsils the size of Jupiter's moons.

Dr. Cyrus puts Kate under a high-powered microscope and tsks. "Her ears are chock full of fluid."

I could cry with relief. "If her ears are full of fluid, why have all the other doctors claimed her ears are fine?"

Dr. Cyrus explains. "A drinking glass filled to the top with water can appear empty if you look through the middle. Kate's ears are so full of fluid that a doctor looking through the fluid might have mistaken her ears as being clear."

Every part of my mothering instinct knows Dr. Cyrus is different. Nothing else the other doctors told me felt exactly right. This feels right. What a difference a good doctor makes.

Dr. Cyrus returns the scope to the lapel pocket of his white lab coat. "I'd venture to guess she doesn't hear well through all that fluid"—I shake my head—"so I want to give her a comprehensive hearing test." He leads us down the hall to a room that looks like a NASA control center. There are no padded earphones from the 1970s or hints of finger rubbing techniques like other doctors have done. The attendant helps Kate step into a soundproof booth and instructs her to raise either hand when she hears a beep, music, or spoken words.

Kate stands perfectly still and watches me through the glass, eager to perform well on this test. Outside the booth, I can also hear the sounds. Instinctively my arms flinch with each beep. Kate flinches her arms when I do, then stops herself from raising her hand all the way, just as I do. She is looking at me for guidance because she can't hear any of the sounds that are wildly beeping, buzzing, and bouncing all around her. Unable to prevent myself from flinching, I finally have to fold my arms tightly across my chest. Like a mirror image, Kate folds her little arms across her chest and waits for my next cue.

The tears surface until I'm watching her through blurred vision. While she hears nothing, I hear the echoes of a hundred interactions with Kate. All the times when my voice would crescendo with anger and impatience… "Why do you always choose to ignore me?" I would grab her little elbow and jerk her around to look into my fiery eyes. "Why do I have to repeat everything ten times to you?" The face she would look into accuses her of being an obstinate, disobedient girl.

I have been yelling at her for years, trying to make her listen. She has spent the same amount of time trying to hear.

There is no tissue in the lab. I hold up a one-minute sign signaling to Kate that I'll be right back. Her face is innocent behind the glass wall. She understands my gesture perfectly. She has become an expert at reading gestures and facial expressions behind soundproof glass. As I walk out of the room, my heart twists on itself with the realization that every time I'd gotten to the point of using gestures to communicate with my daughter, I was already way past patient, far beyond angry and the gestures she saw from me were flailing arms, madly flashing eyes, wide-mouthed beratings. In her short six years of life, this is the communication she has had from me.

ON THE DRIVE home, I explain for Kate what a tonsillectomy and ear tubes mean, but all she wants to know is if she did a good job on the test. Before pulling into the driveway I park in front of our mailbox and reach for the stack of envelopes, advertisements, and newspapers—all things to add on my to-do list.

When we open the front door, Jack pulls his chubby legs under him, sitting up with a self-satisfied grin, and waves for the first time. Kate tugs on my hand. I look down into her soft face and see traces of her baby cheeks.

"Mommy, when they cut my throat and my blood bleeds out, how will the doctors put all the blood back inside?"

The swallow sticks hard in my throat. I should wrap Kate in a reassuring embrace. I should scoop Jack in my arms. I should go through the house gathering all my little people under my wing like a mother hen and apologize for always being so stressed and angry, for always harping about messy rooms and sticky door handles.

"Kate, you won't bleed out all your blood. You'll hardly bleed at all. Go get started on your homework. I'll be right back." The words stutter out more choked than spoken as I turn and escape out the front door, leaving Jack waiting for me to acknowledge his achievement.

The sun is beautiful, the sky a clear blue. The winter grass is brilliant green, the petunias in full bloom. At the time we signed papers to buy this house, I had fallen drunk in love with the idea of eating breakfast as a family on the front porch. Cynthia even left her patio set for us. Today the glass-topped patio table is coated in dirt. I toss the mail on the table and drop into a wrought-iron chair. My elbows smear two dust circles on the glass as my head hangs cumbrous in my hands. We haven't eaten a meal here since…I can't remember.

One by one I pick up the envelopes and toss each aside until I come to a letter addressed to me from the Superior Court of Arizona.

My finger slides under the lip, breaking the seal, and pulls out a crisply folded paper with neatly typed words summoning me for jury duty.

Laiah arrives and joins me at the table. She places a note on top of the mail and points for me to read it. She has designed a clever image—a smiley face with dollar signs for eyes—to tape on my bathroom mirror, a reminder of my goal to boost ad revenue this month by $1,300. I put the note on the tossed-aside pile and lean heavier onto one arm.

"I think I'm going to call a regular doctor." I test the idea on Laiah. By regular doctor, I mean a physician other than my OB-GYN. Naturally anyone in Dr. Woods' office is going to jump to the conclusion of postpartum depression.

"Who is your regular doctor?" Laiah asks.

That's the problem. Outside of my obstetrician, I don't have a doctor. I take my babies to every prenatal appointment before birth and every well child visit after birth. Once they grow teeth, I take them to the dentist every six months, but outside of baby-related issues, I don't have a doctor to check up on the rest of me. Still, sitting here with Laiah, I struggle to know if I'm sick *enough* to merit seeing a doctor.

Holding the letter up again, I study the instructions for reporting to jury duty. The state of Arizona wants me to sit in a courtroom listening to evidence against one of my peers, but I am unfit to judge when the proof is stacked high against *me*. We can't continue living this way. I'm constantly harping at the kids, competing with Aaron, always running behind. For the past weeks Aaron has had to abandon his work to buckle Jack and Tanner in car seats and drive me to my appointments in Goodyear, pulling in front of businesses so I have only a few steps to walk in order to deliver ad proofs. Then he stays awake late working in the office to catch up. Something has to change.

Taking Kate to a new ear, nose, and throat doctor today made all the difference. Instead of looking past her apparently clear but liquid-filled ears, and pronouncing her hearing perfectly fine (when we all knew she was deafer than a post), Dr. Cyrus had gotten to the core of the problem. This is what I need—the right doctor who will look beyond my seven-month-old baby and treat me as a whole person, not just the childbearing parts.

Pulling a random name out of the phone book seems a too-risky version of doctor roulette. Tracing letters of the alphabet into dust on the table, I suddenly remember that years ago—shortly after we'd moved to Surprise—Aaron had gone to someone named Dr. Thorpe. He had impressed me as being intelligent and attentive, someone I could trust. In addition, he is a member of my same church and likely has pioneer ancestors who walked alongside my pioneer ancestors traversing the United States in covered wagons to settle the west. Dr. Thorpe would know it's not in my DNA to complain about a few aches and pains and a bit of the baby blues. He would understand how I'm not bred to quit pushing the handcart before reaching the top of the hill.

So it's Dr. Thorpe's office number I'm seeking when I go inside the house and pull a kitchen chair into the pantry to fetch the yellow pages off the highest shelf. Taking the phone from its cradle, I punch in the number. "Hi, my name is Maleah Warner and I'm calling to make an appointment."

"What seems to be the problem?" The voice on the other end sounds overworked and two hours past due for a break.

I swallow down a big lump of doubt. "I haven't been feeling well…"

Pause.

"Okay…" The voice hints that a little more information could be helpful.

"I'm really tired. Quite often I feel lightheaded…" I can hear her eyes roll so I add, "And my arms get tingly or they go numb."

"What's your date of birth?"

I tell her.

"We don't have you in our system."

"I've never been in before." The answer spills out and too late I realize by the sinking feeling in my stomach that I've solved her dilemma of what to do with me.

"Dr. Thorpe isn't accepting new patients," she says smugly.

"Really?" My voice cracks on the second syllable. I almost hang up the phone, then in desperation I spurt out, "My husband is a patient. Could I set an appointment for him and come in his place?"

"It doesn't work that way," she sighs.

I stay on the line trying to convince her that they must have appointment space available for Aaron, who is in their system, but will not likely be using any of his fairly allotted appointment time share, so why couldn't I use it? At last she makes some excuse and hangs up, leaving me listening to the dial tone.

THAT NIGHT AARON is working late in the office while I lie alone in bed, exhausted but unable to sleep. Pulling off the comforter, I wander into the office wrapped like a mummy and sink to the floor next to Aaron's chair.

"What's up?" he asks.

I don't know how to put it into words other than to say, "I feel a*wful*."

Aaron spreads the comforter on the floor, dims the light, turns on relaxing music, and stretches out next to me so we are face to face.

"I called Dr. Thorpe's office today."

Aaron tries not to look surprised. "When are you going in?"

"I'm not. He isn't taking new patients."

We lie there, two grown-ups, stretched out on our office floor listening to music. Aaron rubs my face and back until I can relax. I think about how much time lately I've spent on floors.

ON SUNDAY EVENING, Aaron returns home from church meetings. "You'll never believe who I bumped into tonight." He tells me he saw Dr. Thorpe and when Dr. Thorpe asked about his family, he mentioned me being sick and that he's worried but doesn't know what to do. "I told him you called his office and got turned down. He said to call his office Monday and he'll get you in."

CHAPTER 32

Sick Enough

TISSUE PAPER CRINKLES under me as I shift uncomfortably on the exam table. My main hope is that I'm sick *enough* to justify Dr. Thorpe finagling his schedule to accommodate me. I'm holding out for a *real* medical diagnosis, not *postpartum depression*—which isn't a medical diagnosis as much as a character assessment revealing a woman of feeble fortitude failing to cope with the normal rigors of motherhood.

"What will you say to Dr. Thorpe?" Laiah quizzed me in preparation. We rehearsed this appointment and tested different dialogue. One problem is that I don't look sick. Nothing on me is broken, swollen, bruised or bleeding. There are no unusual bumps, rashes, or cuts for a doctor to examine. Nothing to x-ray. On the outside I look perfectly fine. In order for Dr. Thorpe to take me seriously and not perceive me as a raging hypochondriac, I've prepared a notebook with two pages listing my symptoms and questions. (This hint came from an article I read entitled "Be Your Own Health Advocate.")

When the doctor enters the room, my hope sinks. It isn't Dr. Thorpe at all. A physician's assistant I've never met reaches out to shake my hand. "I'm Bart Hansen. You can call me Bart. What brings you in today?"

This scene was pre-enacted last night in my mind with Dr. Thorpe playing the role of "ideal medical expert." Gathering my bearings, I do my best to adjust for the change, look at my notes, and begin listing symptoms. "Unexplained weight loss. I'm down to 115 pounds. My clothes don't fit, and my wedding ring slides off my finger. I'm always hungry…"

Bart tilts his head. A woman complaining about being able to eat like a lion and still lose weight? I shouldn't have started with that one. I can almost hear women across the world pleading with me to *please* contaminate them with the same disease, to which I would answer, "Trust me, ladies, you don't want it."

Looking down, I fumble with my notes hoping he will forget about the weight loss comment and forge ahead. "Extreme fatigue. Zero energy. It's so hard to get out of bed and get moving in the morning."

Bart raises his eyebrows like *This lady on the table can't be for real.* None of what I'm saying comes close to describing how rotten I feel. Time to shift gears to things that sound more medical. "I have shakiness, numbness, and tingling in my arms, hands, and sometimes in my legs."

Bart nods, but I can't get a reading on his thoughts.

"Blurry vision. Lightheadedness. Sometimes I get a tin or metallic taste in my mouth. I've been experiencing a decrease in motor skills, like a weak grip and loss of coordination. Also a sore, itchy throat with a lot of drainage and mucus in my chest. I've had a cough all winter that won't go away."

"Are you getting enough sleep?"

I think back to last night, awake until 1:00 a.m. thinking about this appointment, then shortly after dozing off Jack woke up to eat. "I have a hard time falling asleep, and since Christmas my baby has been waking up at night to eat…" The word *baby* spills out of my mouth before I can stop it, so I try to blow past, hoping Bart isn't really listening. "But even if I do sleep a full eight hours, I don't feel any better. Sleep doesn't make a difference in how I feel." How can I convey to this stranger that I am a tough girl? I'm not prone to call a doctor over a few hours of lost sleep and a fuzzy head.

"How old is your baby?"

"Eight months tomorrow," I barely whisper.

Bart snaps his laptop shut. I look down, already knowing what he's going to say. "You know"—he looks at me in a way that tells me I should have known better—"it does take a full twelve months for a woman to completely recover from childbirth."

My body jolts as if something heavy dropped. A surge of frustration boils up until I want to grab Bart by the shirt collar, put my face in his and shout, "Look in these eyes. They are different from your eyes because I am a mother and even my retinas have evolved through the stages of metamorphosis unique to a mother. I see things in microscopic detail that non-mothers miss." Twisting his collar, I would spit into his mouth, "I have had four more babies than you ever will and I am telling you, this time something is different!"

But he's the one with the medical degree, so I sit quietly, hands on my lap, lips closed, grateful he didn't say postpartum depression.

At the door he turns around. "I'll order some blood work…just in case."

A nurse comes in and draws my blood, filling three or four vials with the dark liquid. "How old is your baby?" she chatters away while I bleed into glass. "Oh, that's so fun." She bubbles at the thought of playing mommy. "I don't have children yet, but I want to." She tapes a wad of cotton into the crook of my elbow. "We're all done with you."

At the checkout station, my head hangs while the office manager looks at my chart. "Let's see. You pay one hundred percent of every appointment until you meet your deductible."

Aaron and I pray every day that we'll never meet our $10,000 deductible.

"That will be $125. How do you want to pay?"

In the waiting room, Laiah sits in a leather chair reading *Cosmopolitan*. She looks exactly like the celebrity model on the cover.

Riding down the elevator, I replay the appointment for her. "Basically, I wasted fifteen minutes of Bart's precious time and made a fool of Aaron."

Laiah makes a clicking sound. "One hundred and twenty-five dollars to be told that it takes twelve months to recover from giving birth? You should have gone shopping for shoes.

CHAPTER 33

EBV

MY LAST HOPE is that the blood tests will reveal something to validate why I feel so awful. The days pass, but Dr. Thorpe's office doesn't call with results.

"Maybe they don't call if there's nothing to report," Laiah suggests.

Aaron takes a few more afternoons to drive me to meet customers, then he stops offering. Not only does it interrupt Tanner and Jack's nap schedules and prevent Aaron from finishing his work, but also— though Aaron never admits this out loud—my countenance calls to mind the lead character from *Zombie Bride.* My voice sounds like strained pasta left out to dry, so rather than building good business rapport, I am what the media would call a "public relations nightmare" for our struggling magazine. Perhaps Aaron will grow so annoyed with me that he'll drive me out to the desert and drop me off like an unwanted cat. Part of me wishes he would. I'm no kind of mother and an even lousier excuse for a wife. Each day is a reminder of the worthless human I've become.

The next week Aaron has another unplanned encounter with Dr. Thorpe in the hallway after a seminary meeting. At home, he repeats their conversation for me. "I told him we hadn't heard any results from the blood tests and he was surprised his nurse hadn't called us."

Dr. Thorpe had grabbed Aaron's shoulder and said, "Her blood tests showed a couple of things." According to Aaron, Dr. Thorpe looked serious when he said, "No wonder she feels awful."

"What does she have?" Aaron had asked, somewhat panicked.

"I need to run more tests before I have definitive answers. Call my office tomorrow and schedule a follow-up," Dr. Thorpe had said then left Aaron staring and hurried off to another meeting.

In bed Aaron sleeps soundly while I lie awake mulling over Dr. Thorpe's statement. *Her blood tests showed a couple of things.* My eyes watch the odd shapes of night shadows move stealthily across the ceiling. A car engine turns over at the neighbor's house. The words churn in my head: *No wonder she feels so awful.*

There is a reason, then—a cause behind my inability to function? Dr. Thorpe's words give me hope of validation, the possibility that I'm not a weak woman, but a strong woman dealing with a *real* physical challenge. But what did my blood tests show? The possibilities are numerous. I could stay awake exploring them most of the night, which I do, counting the potential maladies higher than numbers of sheep, at last falling asleep to the gentle lullaby of those liberating words: *No wonder she feels so awful*—a phrase which to me carries the relief and freedom of what a courtroom defendant must feel upon hearing the declaration *not guilty.*

—◦◦◦—

BEFORE THE END of the week I'm wearing another hospital gown (cloth this time) while Nadine, the ultrasound technician, smears warm jelly up and down my neck. *What is she looking for? A tumor? Cancer?*

"Do you see anything suspicious, Nadine?" My chin is pointed high while she presses the probe deep against my jugular vein, clicking a button to capture images.

"We're not allowed to say anything." Nadine clicks the mouse with a perfect poker face, highlighting secret numbers and codes around the black and white detail of my thyroid on the monitor. "Your doctor will give you the results."

Without moving my neck, my eyes strain to spy if her fingers type the letters c-a-n-c-e-r. After a week of researching possible ailments from myelinolysis to meningitis, the conclusion I've drawn is that thyroid cancer is the ideal malady. Thyroid cancer is a serious enough diagnosis to prove that this is not a weak character issue. Also, the appearance of the word *cancer* in any form immediately garners attention and sympathy and basically comes with a doctor's excuse note to skip out on life responsibility for a while:

Dear World,

Excuse Maleah from any obligations. She has cancer. Give her nonjudgmental permission to stay in bed while you watch her children. Give her your sympathy and deliver warm casseroles at 5:00 each evening. Do not ask her to spearhead the school carnival this year.

Sincerely,
God

Is it wrong, this morbid sense of satisfaction at being able to "stick it" to all the people who haven't believed me? My mind paints a gratifying picture of a guilt-ridden Bart Hansen tossing and turning in bed and promising, "I'll never speak in a condescending way to any mother who comes into my office, ever again."

A diagnosis of thyroid cancer would mean people rallying to my aid. Aaron will hold my hand and watch me with worried eyes, apologizing that he insisted we go to Utah for Christmas. Bob will tell me I've worked too hard and not to worry about the magazine. My brothers will send flowers. My mom and sister will arrive to clean my house. Ladies at church will bring dinner and volunteer to watch the kids.

Laiah agrees that thyroid cancer is the optimal outcome. "It will bring you sympathy, apology, and vindication. You deserve all that."

In the end, my diagnosis will be exactly what I deserve.

—⟋⟍⟋—

"GREAT NEWS!" DR. Thorpe breezes into the exam room. "Your thyroid looks fantastic. No lumps, growths, or lesions." Dr. Thorpe appears pleased to deliver good news, then his smile drops, and he looks puzzled as my expression changes from hopeful anticipation to disappointment. A clean ultrasound pulls the rug out of my mandatory hospital vacation. What about, *No wonder she feels so awful?*

"So, what *is* wrong with me?" I can't go home emptyhanded. What could I say to Aaron, to Bob, to people at church, to my family... that the doctor couldn't find anything wrong with me so it must be all in my head?

"One of the blood tests we ran was an Epstein-Barr titer. You've had Epstein-Barr for over eight weeks."

"What is Epstein-Barr?" The term is recognizable, though I've always heard Epstein-Barr tossed into the same hat as chronic fatigue and fibromyalgia—a vague category of illnesses that doctors assign names to so they don't have to tell patients, "We don't know what's wrong with you." These are the types of illnesses that label a person as "sick" with questionable air quotation marks. Of all the thousands of possible outcomes I'd envisioned, not one scenario had remotely considered the possibility of a mystery illness, one that comes with a lifetime warranty and no cure.

Dr. Thorpe gives a medical school explanation about how a few different viruses are known to have only one nucleus and thus merit the name *mono*nucleosis, so the "knock you down, make you ultra-tired" illness that society commonly refers to as "mono" isn't the only *mono*nucleic virus. This microbiology lesson doesn't make me any wiser regarding my condition.

"So, do I have mono?" I ask for clarification.

"The Epstein-Barr virus can cause mono, but it can cause other illnesses, too." Dr. Thorpe flips over the printout of my lab numbers and draws a graph. "All we really know is that eight weeks ago your immune system created antibodies against the Epstein-Barr virus."

Eight weeks ago, I left urgent care with an antibiotic prescription for strep throat, but since the lab technician was gone, they hadn't swabbed my throat to make certain. "Can mono or Epstein-Barr symptoms be confused with strep throat?"

"Some of the symptoms of mono are similar to strep throat such as coughing, mucus buildup, and extreme fatigue." Having delivered his good news about my thyroid, Dr. Thorpe closes his laptop, ready to move through the lineup of patients waiting for him. His waiting room had been crowded, but I'm still confused.

"What about my thyroid?" I'm desperate for more answers.

"Your TSH, or thyroid stimulating hormone, was high the first time, but this last test came back at 3.2, which is well within normal range. It's possible that the EBV had thrown your thyroid temporarily out of whack."

Dr. Thorpe starts to leave again, but I don't know what step to take next. What do I go home and tell Aaron?

"Wait. I still have some questions, if that's okay?"

Dr. Thorpe leans against the counter as I open my red notebook and fire a volley of questions at him: "Could the surge in my thyroid number be a sign of a deeper problem? Did the tests definitively rule out a tumor or cancer? Are there other tests I should get? Why do I have trouble falling asleep at night? What can I do about the coughing and the phlegm? How can I be sure I don't have something more serious?"

Dr. Thorpe gives short answers, hinting that my fifteen-minute appointment with him is over.

"Am I contagious?" I'm thinking about all the poor people who've been on the receiving end of one of my hugs, kisses, or handshakes over the past eight weeks—piano recital guests, business contacts, Aaron's family over Christmas, my family who slept at my house and ate the food I'd coughed onto, and Jack—there's no way I haven't exposed Jack.

"If we tested the population, probably ninety percent of adults would already have antibodies to the Epstein-Barr virus, showing that they've been exposed to it at some point in their life. A lot of people don't realize they've had mono; for them it manifests as a cold. And children don't usually get mono."

"How do I get better?"

"There are a couple of new antiviral drugs on the market: one that fights herpes—and the EB virus is related to the herpes virus—but you usually have to take it within three days of the viral onset. Whether it would help against a two-month-old virus is questionable, but you could try." He hands me a prescription for the new, experimental, antiviral medication, and a lab order to re-test my thyroid in six weeks, then leaves me staring at the cotton swabs in the glass jar next to the sink.

AFTER THE APPOINTMENT I call my doctor brother, Paul, for a second opinion. "Those antibodies could be from when you had mono in college. Mono is like chicken pox," he explains. "A person gets mono once, then the immune system develops antibodies so you never get mono again, and the antibodies will stay in your blood and show up on lab tests for the rest of your life."

I hang up the phone more confused than before. Possibly I have mono, possibly I don't. Possibly I have a variant disease caused by the Epstein-Barr virus. Possibly my thyroid isn't working. Possibly my thyroid is working fine. This isn't what I'd expected. I'd wanted a clear diagnosis with a scientific name and no ambiguous connotation that me being "sick" is all in my head.

Should I take the antivirals?

The pharmacy is lined with ceramic planter pots overflowing with thick petunia plants sporting jumbo red and white blossoms. This has been an especially good winter for petunias, even the petunias in my own planter boxes boast larger petals than I've ever seen. Opening the glass door, I face my own wilted reflection—everything around here is thriving except for me.

While the pharmacist fills the prescription, I roam the infant care aisle debating which brand of formula to use for Jack. The antivirals haven't been on the market long enough to prove safe for breastfeeding. The decision has been made for me—I will be weaning Jack.

Aaron greets me at the front door rocking a hungry Jack in his arms. He leans in to kiss me, his breath on my cheek feels bated. Perhaps he's been waiting for the results of this appointment with nerves as anxious as my own. "What did Dr. Thorpe say?"

And so it begins. Aaron is the first in a lineup of people who will ask what the doctor found. My decision to take the antivirals probably had more to do with having an answer to their questions than out of belief they would make a difference.

"He said I have a virus. He put me on an antiviral medication."

Yes, this is the answer I will give them all, from my siblings to the ladies at church: "Doctor says it's a virus, I'm taking an *antiviral*." Which is so much different than saying, "Doctor says it's depression. I'm taking an *antidepressant*."

Aaron seems relieved. Carrying Jack to Breastfeeding Basecamp, I smother his ear, neck and cheeks with kisses. Dr. Thorpe said babies can't get mono. "Are you starving, little man?" I lift my shirt and let him nurse for as long as he wants—or at least as long as it takes for me to stop crying. Later that afternoon, when I give Jack his first bottle of infant formula, he looks into my eyes with curious satisfaction as if to say, "So this is what real nutrition tastes like. What took you so long?"

That afternoon Aaron moves Jack's crib out of our bedroom. I cross my heart, spit into my palm, and shake hands promising Aaron that for one week I will let Jack cry during the night instead of getting up to comfort or feed him. It's about time we all start sleeping through the night.

CHAPTER 34

Waiting Game

DR. THORPE'S *GET Well* plan is more like a six-week round of the Waiting Game: take the antivirals, wait for the virus to pass, come back in six weeks for a follow-up thyroid blood test.

Before the appointment, I'd convinced myself that Dr. Thorpe would give me news along the lines of "You've got a parasitic, energy-zapping tumor wrapped around your thyroid, which explains why you can't move or take a full breath. One little outpatient surgery and you will be good as new!"

What I had expected was a scenario similar to my Lasik eye surgery two years ago. On that day I walked into the doctor's office with vision so blurry I could barely decipher the large E on top of the eye charts. One hour later, driving home from the procedure, miniscule letters on road signs a mile away were crystal clear. Laiah and I had persuaded ourselves that the one and only possible outcome of the appointment would be Dr. Thorpe sending me for surgery. The surgery would be serious enough to warrant get well cards and warm casseroles delivered from church ladies, but not too risky. Most importantly, during the surgery I would be unconscious while someone other than myself worked to remove the problem and I would wake up *all* better.

But that isn't what happened. I'm not even close to being *all* better. Getting the kids ready in the morning feels like trying to push the bus to school by myself. Our March deadline is looming, and menial tasks take me hours to complete. Aaron speeds past me in the hall as I move slow as a tortoise treading through a river of thick tar. He prepares dinner, feeds the kids and finishes the dishes before I can open the fridge and take out the milk.

How will I get through the next six weeks?

Some days I feel so terrible that I'm convinced I will die. But even worse than the thought of death is the prospect that I won't die, but won't get better either, and will have to clunk through the rest of my life like a zombie on crutches. Which is no life at all.

The monster-sized antiviral capsules remind me of the pills my dad forced down a calf's throat to treat it for scours. Each night before bed I gulp one of those massive pills and hope that come sunrise, my eyes will open and I'll be able to take a full breath and say, "Wow, I feel better." During the day, my body wears a cloak of fatigue, but the moment my body reposes for the night, I come wide awake.

I can*not* fall asleep.

If there is one area in which I've excelled in my life, it is being an accomplished sleeper. Up until now I could fall asleep anywhere: in the car, on my school desk, sitting upright in the pew at church, on the park bench watching my kids swing. Given three minutes of stillness, I could breeze through REM and achieve full nirvana-like sleep. There are plenty of skills I lack (running, for example—I will never be found breaking the ribbon at the end of a race), but if sleeping were an Olympic event, you could pad your bank account betting on me to win consecutive gold medals.

Until now.

Now, I am failing at sleep. This is an entirely new experience for me.

Lying in bed my head itches, so I get up and brush my hair. Back between the sheets my pillow needs re-fluffing. Lying on the right side of my body isn't comfortable, but neither is flipping to the left. An army of a red ants marches up the insides of my legs. My nerves are on fire. In the toss and turn, the covers are pulled off Aaron who sits up irritated. "What are you doing?"

"I can't fall asleep!"

"Why?"

If I knew why I would fix it.

Holding as still as possible so Aaron can sleep, I count seconds, telling myself I must reach three hundred before switching positions, but my skin becomes a scratchy wool blanket. Kicking back the covers and switching on the bright bathroom light, I dig through the under-sink cabinet searching for hydrocortisone or lotion with anti-itch remedy. Rubbing lotion into my dry skin drives the ants away until the moment my feet settle into the bottom of the sheets, then the ants are back, those pesky, determined little skin crawlers. The pillow under my face barely muffles my frustrated screams.

"What is wrong?!" Aaron's patience with me has worn paper thin.

I don't *know* what's wrong! My body is run-down, but instead of being sleepy, my eyes, brain, and circuits are on high alert. I can't stand my bedroom any longer. With a pillow tucked under my arm and a spare blanket from the linen closet in the hall, I set up night watch on the family room couch.

For ten nights I put on pajamas, swallow a massive antiviral pill, crawl into bed, and hope to wake up feeling better. What I crave more than anything is the energy and renewal that come from restorative sleep. For ten mornings I find myself greeting sunrise through the family room window, not refreshed, not rejuvenated, only resentful.

Waking up on yet another morning to find himself alone in bed, Aaron politely suggests that this "trouble sleeping" is all in my head and perhaps I should break the habit of moving to the couch in the night. Mentally, I chain my body to the mattress. Eventually, Aaron falls asleep. My eyes close, the edges of dreams appear to escort my consciousness into sleep. A deep exhale. The first frames of dream are loudly interrupted, a movie reel broken and flapping, the screen white with choppy countdown numbers. I bolt upright and gasp.

What woke me? My ears perk, listening for the sound: Something fell off a kitchen shelf? One of the kids rolled out of bed? An alarm? A police siren? All is silent. The house and yard are peaceful.

Aaron rolls over. "What is it?"

"Did you hear something?"

"No." He nestles back into his pillow. "I didn't hear anything." Without effort, Aaron returns to a soothing pattern of deep, relaxed breathing.

Lying next to his dozing body, I am anything but restful. My pulse races as if I am trying to outrun a bear. I try to return to my dream, but my body and mind—though flattened with fatigue—are wide awake. The clock reads 12:43 a.m. *No getting out of bed!* I tell myself. Like a prisoner paces the boundaries of the jail cell, I toss and turn, pushing against the limited confines of my bed. I roll as far away from Aaron as I can get, but that doesn't help, so I roll over and entwine myself around him, hoping his sleepiness will spread to me. *Don't look at the clock.* Scooting back to the middle of my space, I cross my legs, uncross my legs, change the pillow between my knees, curl into a tight ball, stretch out long and straight, lie on my back, lie on my stomach. *Oops, I looked at the clock*: 2:34 a.m. Two hours and no sleep! My anger flares; I throw off the covers and launch my pillow against the wall, letting out a tribal yell. Aaron opens his eyes to see me pulling my hair as if trying to remove my scalp.

"What is *wrong*?" he asks, propping up onto one elbow.

"I CANNOT SLEEP!" My bottled emotions well up and pop their cork like bitter champagne. "I have not fallen asleep since that first time when something jerked me awake."

"You're kidding. Why?"

"I DON'T KNOW WHY!" There is an overwhelming urge to leap out of bed and pound the walls. Something in me desperately needs to throw a couch. "I want to sleep. I am exhausted, but my body will *not* fall asleep."

Aaron looks incredulous. I hide my head. How does he do it? He makes sleeping look so easy.

Thus I spend my nights, squashed between Fatigue and Insomnia, the unlikeliest of bedfellows. What's more, sometime in the night, a soot-covered, burly blacksmith comes into the room and sets up his cumbersome anvil on my chest. He goes to work pounding and bending his iron—my lungs and ribs crush under his labor. In the wee morning hours, Insomnia grows disenchanted by the noise and exits the room, leaving Fatigue and me huddled together under the weight of the blacksmith's anvil.

———

IN THE MIDST of all this *non*-sleeping, my house becomes Hotel Arizona. Since moving to Surprise seven years ago, our house has been a spring break retreat for friends, cousins, and cousins of our friends' cousins. From March through April, anyone seeking reprieve from the bitter clutches of the northern winter calls to reserve a room at the Warner Bed & Breakfast.

In the past I have loved these visitors who entertain my children and break up the monotony of day-to-day housekeeping. But this year I lack the strength to hold up the two corners of my mouth, let alone carry on congenial conversation. And how will I explain to my guests about the black circles under my eyes?

When my cousin's family comes to stay, she brings a health drink which is supposed to cure everything from toe fungus to a bad personality. Desperate enough to try anything, I take a cautious sip, barely stopping myself from gagging. Does it taste more like what goes into a horse's mouth or what comes out its other end?

"Sorry, it doesn't taste good," she says in sympathy, "but it works really well."

The email I send to one of my favorite visitors takes me an hour to write. I want to see her. We need her humor and sense of pragmatism, not to mention the kids *adore* her. But she's recently been diagnosed with multiple sclerosis and I'm a walking petri dish.

Dear Janyce,

I'm thinking that your compromised immune system and the questionable contagiousness of my possible virus may not be a good combination. Maybe you should keep your distance from me this year.

Maleah

The last visitors who come to town are my parents. After a morning of throwing bread crumbs to ducks at the neighborhood park, we take a scenic tour of every house with a "for sale" sign. At each stop my dad climbs out of the car to retrieve an info sheet, which he adds to the rolled stack of flyers ripping the seams of his shirt pocket. "Honey," he says to my mother, "we ought to buy a home and move down here. I'm getting too old to shovel snow." The moderate March weather casts a spell on people, hypnotizing them into believing they *must* move here, but come July, Hotel Arizona is more hell than heaven.

While we drive, I paraphrase what the doctors said at my two appointments. Mom wonders if I've called for Paul's opinion, which I have. "So basically, nobody knows what is wrong with me, or nothing is wrong with me and it's all in my head."

My dad signals me to stop the car. In talking about my confusing diagnosis, I missed a house for sale. Dad stoops his tall frame back into the minivan, stuffing yet another trifold in his pocket along with the case for his sunglasses. That pocket has exceeded its holding capacity. Resuming the conversation without missing a beat, my dad tells me about a young mother from his church congregation (where he serves as the bishop) who got really sick last year and no one could find out what was wrong with her. "We all thought she was on her deathbed, then she found this one doctor and now she runs around with so much energy you'd never know she was sick."

"What doctor did she go to?" I ask.

My dad thinks hard. "She went to see one of those *homo*...what do you call them? *Homeo*...honey?" He asks my mom for help, but she has no idea what he's talking about. "Homeophobic!" my dad spouts out. "That's it. She went to one of those *homeo*phobic doctors and now she is one hundred percent better."

Though my health status is confusing, I'm confident *homeo*phobia is not my problem; still, the thought of my traditional father suggesting natural medicine raises the corners of my mouth a few degrees. Growing up my parents viewed chiropractors and homeopaths with the same suspicion as fortune tellers and gold diggers.

"You ought to go see one of those *homeo*phobic doctors," my dad tells me. Then again, Dad is always bringing up things people *ought* to do: "Honey, we ought to move down here." Or, "That's a nifty gadget you're using to slice meat. Honey, you ought to get one of those."

THAT EVENING, AFTER my parents leave for Annice's house, I drop in to a church women's gathering. I didn't feel up to going, but Mom had said, "You should go. Those meetings are always so good. I ought to stay and go with you, but we told Annice we would come for dinner."

When the meeting ends, some of the ladies gather to talk. They end up circled around me, not because I am the life of the party but because I couldn't muster the strength to move.

Laura says, "Maleah, you're looking good tonight."

This is what comes out of my mouth and I'm not proud about it: "There's a reason they put makeup on dead people."

Lately I am fun to be around in the way a barrel of decaying monkeys is fun. In response to my snarky comment, these ladies have every right to fold their metal chairs and leave me to my self-pity. Instead, they gather closer.

"What's up, Maleah? What's going on?" Deanne asks.

Surprising myself, I open up about the diagnosis or non-diagnosis. "I'm getting worse and I don't know how to get better."

Hannah says, "Go see Dr. Erdmann."

Crystal pipes in, "Yes. Go see Dr. Erdmann."

"What does he do?" I ask.

"He's a homeopathic doctor."

"Yeah, but what does he *do*?" I have no experience with homeopathic doctors.

"Just go see him and find out what he thinks," Hannah says.

"That's interesting, my dad said the same thing to me this morning." I look around realizing we are the last people in the meeting room. These women will be late getting home to babies and husbands. They have stayed late to rally around me.

CHAPTER 35

Homeophobic

AROUND 1985, GIVE or take a few years, Dr. Anderson opened the first chiropractic clinic in my hometown. When Mother spied someone we knew opening his office door, she would say, "Now why are *they* going in *there*?" as if the person were walking into a house of ill repute. People entering the state liquor store didn't get the same height of my mother's eyebrows as people visiting the chiropractor.

And now I have an appointment with one.

Flying to Tanzania and climbing Mt. Kilimanjaro to speak to a guru might feel less absurd. For three days I've tried to visualize the appointment and for some reason these imaginations always show Dr. Erdmann as a burly, bearded man who lives in a trailer in the desert and eats roasted lizards and cactus juice. Also, he has three albino snakes. On my way to the appointment, I wonder if this will be a traditional question-and-answer type exam, or will there be bloodletting leeches?

The address takes me to a newly built office complex. The lettering on the clear glass door reads *Dr. Robert Erdmann, D.C.* On the waiting room table is a stack of magazines—the typical, run-of-the-mill reading selections—none of which promote a Himalayan mud diet.

A receptionist hands me a clipboard. "Welcome. I'm Julia. Since this is your first visit, please fill out these forms." Pulling a flower pen from the jar of flat marbles, I take a seat in the far corner and speak a silent, in-my-head kind of prayer. *Please let me know if this doctor can help me.* I need divine enlightenment to sort out if this homeopathic mumbo-jumbo merits an investment of my time and money or if the whole setup is a shenanigan my brother Paul likes to call "a lot of hocus pocus." A warmth spreads in my chest. It feels right to be here.

The top forms are the standard insurance information and privacy disclosures, but the next form is different. Rather than mindlessly checking boxes about family history of diabetes and arthritis, these questions probe deeper.

List your symptoms in order of what is most disruptive to your life.

SLEEP: I feel so weary and worn down, but I can't sleep!

It's oddly touching that someone wants to understand how the ailments that bring me in today are impeding my day-to-day quality of life. Writing out "I can't sleep!" in real letters on tangible paper is empowering. Without even seeing Dr. Erdmann, my body feels buoyed up, as if I'm Atlas struggling to hold the weight of my world and someone put a support beam under my arm. This is the right doctor for me. The flower pen moves across the page and the rest of my symptoms appear, written evidence to issues I've worried were all in my head.

Lightheaded: I'm scared to drive long distances. I feel like I don't exist, like there is no substance to me.

Muddy head: Forgetfulness. Can't make decisions or solve problems. It's hard to feel intuition or inspiration like before.

Congestion/cough: Lots of sinus drainage and chest muck.

Aches: Feels like the worst body aches from flu every day.

Slow: I move slowly and don't get things done like I used to.

Hormones: Anxiousness and rage. I feel ready to explode, even when I'm not mad at anything, but I don't feel other emotions like happy or sad.

Weakness: No strength. I have nothing to offer. I don't feel any weight on my feet, no foundation. Worthless.

Wellness: No sense of wellness. I can feel that something is wrong with me, but I can't tell what it is.

Only very last do I write:

Tingling/numbness in my arms and legs.

The tingling is what I emphasized to Bart Hansen, not that it bothers me the most, because it doesn't, but because it seemed the most likely to merit medical concern. The inability to sleep, the muddy head, and the body aches didn't seem like something worth seeing a doctor about, yet they are the very things that most disrupt my daily ability to function.

A nurse opens the door and calls my name. I follow her through the door, taking the first step of a thousand-mile journey.

DR. ERDMANN BREEZES into the room with giant strides on short legs. He looks like a five-foot-six weightlifter and wears—of all the bizarre things—Dockers and a polo shirt.

"Hey! How ya doing?" He grins with so much enthusiasm I think maybe he ended up with my energy and I only needed to come here today to reclaim it.

Without looking at my paperwork, he proceeds to do what, I later learn, is called muscle testing. He taps on different places around my back and belly, asking questions and pushing on my outstretched arm. Sometimes my arm stays firm and sometimes my arm drops like a lever. Next, he pulls out a silver briefcase and sets it on his lap. Dr. Erdmann snaps the latches which make a double *click, click*. With a *you're going to love this* smile, he raises the lid.

Part of me expects him to lift out a .44 Remington Magnum with a three-inch silencer. Yes, the environment feels that far from my "normal," and yet, I don't feel uncomfortable. Okay, maybe I feel a little uncomfortable.

The suitcase, though cushioned with felt, is not housing pistol, but vials of glass specimen jars holding samples of what look like pieces of lint, dirt, some metal shavings, colored solutions, and pills. He holds various vials up to different parts of my body and does the same arm pushing. He talks so fast I can't follow everything he says. Suddenly the vials are all returned to their foam resting spots. The suitcase is snapped shut and stashed under the counter.

"Take a seat." Dr. Erdmann gestures for me to sit on the examination table. "You have a virus in your spleen. Your spleen is quite swollen."

One of the tests Dr. Thorpe had ordered was an ultrasound of my spleen. I didn't mention spleen anywhere on my paperwork. *Weird.* Was he a chiropractor...or a *fortune teller*?

Dr. Erdmann continues. "You also have an infection, but what puzzles me the most is"—he presses into my lower back—"have you done something to burn out your adrenal glands?"

"Have I what?"

"Burned out your adrenal glands. You've heard about adrenaline rushes?"

Sure, I've heard miracle stories about the mother who lifts a car off her child or the man who outruns a flash flood, feats of extreme strength or speed coming from a boost of adrenaline.

"The fight or flight response is designed to be a quick, short-term reaction to survive an extreme circumstance. After the emergency, the body must rest in order to rebuild and restore its adrenal function." Dr. Erdmann crosses his arms and tsk-tsks like a school principal trying to decide what to do with a naughty student. "Your adrenal glands are torched, like you've been burning through adrenaline over an extended period of time."

"Umm. Last fall I helped clean out my parents' house. There were a lot of heavy boxes, fifty pound buckets of wheat, and I moved furniture like beds and dressers..." Pictures flash through my mind: bracing a heavy wooden chest of drawers with my nephew balancing the other end while we struggled to heft it up the concrete stairs out of the basement. After two days of emptying the house, I returned straight to teaching early-morning seminary. Then I was pregnant, and the magazine...the drive to Tucson, the bath, the lights, the commotion of Jack's frantic birth, his blessing—the images flash by in microseconds, but I seem to relive each and every event including my midnight visit with Amanda, the visit to urgent care, my final piano recital, traveling for Christmas, hosting my family for New Year's, the Chamber of Commerce presentation...

"I might have..."

"Come back in two days." He hands me a paper and leaves the room.

At the front desk Julia takes my paper and gathers bottles of supplements off a shelf. "The appointment is forty dollars and the supplements add up to"—she types numbers into a calculator—"ninety-five dollars."

Dr. Erdmann had spent an hour with me and actually examined my body. Unlike Dr. Thorpe, who had sat at a distance and asked questions, Dr. Erdmann had probed, adjusted, snapped things back into place, giving the impression he was cleaning house, clearing clutter and putting things back in order. The whole appointment including supplements totaled $135—nearly the same cost as one fifteen-minute office visit to Dr. Thorpe. My insurance doesn't cover naturopathy or *homeophoby* or whatever you call what Dr. Erdmann does, so at the front desk I pay for the appointment with $150 in cash received from returning gifts to the store. Julia accepts the bills. "Would you like credit or change?"

Her question strikes me in a new way. I look up, tilting my head, feeling a subtle *click*. "I want...*change*."

"Dr. Erdmann wants to see you again Thursday. How about 12:15?"

"Fine," I answer, still stunned.

On the walk out to my car, the cells in my body seem to raise their hands in a unanimous vote: "Yes. This is what we need. Please bring us back."

At home Aaron fixes lunch while I rattle on about the arm pushing, the silver briefcase full of mystery vials, the torched adrenals.

"Wow, that is weird. How do people believe in that stuff?" He laughs. I don't laugh with him. He notices my sober expression. "You were joking, right? Oh, you're not joking. You're serious about this?"

"I wish you could have been there in person. What he said made sense. He gave me a lot more answers than Dr. Thorpe. Retelling makes it sound like voodoo magic."

"You sound like you're going back."

"I have another appointment on Thursday."

CHAPTER 36

Hashimoto's

AFTER VISITING DR. Erdmann two or three times a week over the past month, I've come to expect the unexpected. Each session is a surprise—everything from color therapy to acupuncture. On one visit he took me to a back room and instructed his assistant to prepare a foot bath. "These foot baths use positive or negative ionic charges to draw toxins out of the body. Your body is full of thallium. Strange, we usually see thallium in people who have worked in coal mines or coal-burning power plants." Dr. Erdmann put a metal rod into the water with my feet. "We'll start you with twenty minutes today and work up little by little."

He flipped on a switch and I flinched, expecting an electric shock, but there was no shock, only soothing warm water. I relaxed and leaned back in the chair, certain that I'd never mentioned growing up near coal mines and power plants to Dr. Erdmann.

The water remained clear for five minutes then—out from the bottoms of my feet—clouds of yellow muck started to form. *What in the world?* The yellow clouds floated to the surface and were followed by a brown, gravy-like goop. More minutes passed and green mixed with the brown and yellow. Next, flecks of what looked like colored metallic shavings floated to the top.

After twenty minutes, Dr. Erdmann returned to check on me.

"It looks disgusting," I said, watching the swirl of filth around my ankles.

"It's not the worst I've seen," Dr. Erdmann replied. "I've had patients who turned the water black the first time." Dr. Erdmann bent down and pointed. "See this foam? That is mucus from your chest."

My eyes popped open wide and I leaned for a closer look. All the phlegm I'd been coughing up! The nagging cough and congestion had been number four on symptoms that most disrupted my life, but I'd never verbally addressed the issue to Dr. Erdmann. Either this ion thingy really did work or Dr. Erdmann had been studying my paperwork and catering his hocus pocus to my unique symptoms. In either case, I was impressed with his attentiveness.

At home Aaron listened as I animatedly described the foot baths. "That sounds like bogus science," he said.

"It makes sense to me. Everything else in life requires regular cleaning and maintenance—the house, car, yard, jacuzzi. Why not the body?" The idea of pulling out trash that has been collecting in my systems felt intuitively right to me. I wished I could go back and ask Dr. Erdmann for a sample of my foot water to bring home so Aaron would believe me.

―――⌕⌕⌕――――

SEVERAL WEEKS LATER and at last it's time for my six-week follow-up visit with Dr. Thorpe. There is almost a skip in my step walking through his waiting room to sign in for the appointment. Won't Dr. Thorpe be pleased about the amazing answers Dr. Erdmann has given me? My red notebook is bulging with the questions and information I've gathered in the time since we last met. I anticipate the three of us working together—Dr. Thorpe, Dr. Erdmann, and myself—will make a fine team to solve my health conundrum. After today's appointment, Dr. Thorpe will be on board, then Aaron will come around.

My pen and notebook are open and ready when Dr. Thorpe knocks and enters. "I've made some progress since my last appointment,"

I say right off the bat. "I've done research and I've been visiting Dr. Erdmann." Dr. Thorpe nods, indicating he knows about Dr. Erdmann. "He says I have adrenal fatigue." I announce the news as if the mystery has been solved at last!

Dr. Thorpe shakes his head, and suddenly I know he's heard this line a hundred times before. "Adrenal fatigue is not a medical diagnosis. There is something called Addison's disease where your adrenals don't function at all."

"Did you get the results of my blood cortisol tests that Dr. Erdmann requested?"

"Yes. Your levels are within normal range." Dr. Thorpe hands me a copy.

"My cortisol level was sixteen and the normal range is from twelve to sixty-four? I'm on the low end. Do you think I should be tested for Addison's?"

"If you had Addison's, you wouldn't have been able to walk in here."

I wanted to point out that I could barely walk in here. This appointment is not going how I anticipated. I hoped when Dr. Thorpe jumped on the homeopathic bandwagon, that Aaron would be soon to follow.

Dr. Thorpe continues, "About your thyroid…"

"Yes. I have some questions." I flip through my notebook to find the page with my thyroid research. "I read there's something called postnatal hypothyroid where a woman can be hypothyroid for a while after giving birth, but over time her thyroid naturally goes back to normal function. That would explain why I haven't felt good after some of my other babies." I'm hoping he will come to the same conclusion, that my thyroid malfunction was a temporary issue.

"Your second thyroid blood test showed that you have Hashimoto's Thyroiditis." Dr. Thorpe lays his trump card on the table.

"What?" I have no idea what he just said.

"Hashimoto's Thyroiditis causes you to be hypothyroid. It means your own immune system has produced antibodies that are attacking your thyroid."

"How come that didn't show up on the first test?"

"The first time we only tested for TSH levels. The second test I ordered was specifically to test for anti-TPO antibodies, which you do have." He speed-talks through an explanation of the presence of anti-thyroid peroxidase indicating an autoimmune disease.

"But what does that *mean?*" The sudden change of direction has thrown me off-kilter.

"Eventually your thyroid will burn out." Dr. Thorpe shows me a copy of my lab numbers and I notice the date of the results are four weeks old.

I drop my notebook in my lap. "How does a person live with a dead thyroid?"

"You take medication. I'd start you on fifty micrograms of Synthroid. You take one pill every morning on an empty stomach and get your TSH blood levels tested every few months. Over time, you'll incrementally increase your dose until the medicine completely replaces what the thyroid used to do."

"For the rest of my life?"

"There's no way to stop it. Eventually your own immune system will destroy your thyroid. Whether this takes one year or twenty years, there's no way to tell."

I don't want my thyroid to burn out. I never paid much attention to the little gland before and suddenly I regret taking it for granted. "Surely some people get better, don't they?" I ask again sounding skeptical of his conclusions. "If Hashimoto's is autoimmune, that means it can autocorrect, right?"

Dr. Thorpe takes a deep breath. "There's about a ten percent chance your thyroid could recover on its own."

"What if I don't take the medicine? Will I die?"

"You won't die, but you won't feel better unless you take the medicine."

Again with doctors and prescription drugs. Fresh on my mind is what happened two weeks ago after Kate's tonsillectomy.

———⁓———

WE ARRIVED AT Phoenix Children's Hospital at 6:00 a.m. for the operation. About 10:00 the anesthesiologist swung through the door to give me the post-surgery report. He looked like a soap opera doctor, a handsome male model dressed in scrubs pretending to be an anesthesiologist. "It's done. Kate did great. Man, those were the biggest adenoids I've ever seen." He shook his head from astonishment. "You can go wait with her in the recovery room."

When Kate woke up she accepted a popsicle right away.

"You can take her home now anytime you want," said the nurse, handing me a prescription for Tylenol with codeine. "You'll want to fill this prescription on your way home, before the anesthesia wears completely off."

"Isn't codeine a pretty strong drug for a six-year-old?" I questioned. "We hardly take any medicine. Can I start her on regular children's Tylenol and then see if she needs this?"

"My daughter got her tonsils out two weeks ago and she said it was the worst pain she's ever had."

"How old is your daughter?" I asked.

"She's twenty-one."

"Young kids are pretty resilient. They fall down and bounce right back up."

The nurse was insistent. "You're going to want to keep her medicated, stay on top of the pain, or she's going to be very sore."

"Doesn't codeine make you nauseous?" I tried to remember something I'd heard.

"This is what we prescribe to all our kids." She closed her book as if she had the final answer.

Not knowing whether to defer to the hospital's recommended practices or my personal inclination to let the human body heal on its own, I called Aaron to be the tiebreaker. He's always giving the kids cold medicine behind my back when I prefer to let them tough it out, so I mostly called to hear his voice of reassurance that it would be okay to give Kate the prescription meds. Surprisingly, Aaron said, "Tylenol with codeine is pretty strong stuff. I had that when I hurt my back in high school and it knocked me out. I would say bring her home and let's see how she does without it."

At home Kate gobbled down another popsicle and accepted a dose of over-the-counter children's pain relief. By afternoon she was bouncing around with Danny and Tanner.

"Kate, how are you doing?" I asked. "Do you want more medicine?"

"No thanks." She jumped from the couch into the bean bag.

"How does your throat feel?" I prodded.

"It's scratchy, but the popsicles make it feel better," she announced, hopping up from her flip.

"Mom," Danny laughed. "She sounds funny."

If it weren't for her Minnie Mouse voice, we would hardly know she'd had surgery a few hours earlier. From that night on she has slept quiet as a church mouse, no more snoring like a tree-trimmer running a chainsaw.

What happened next is the reason I stall when Dr. Thorpe hands me the Synthroid prescription.

One week after Kate's surgery, my friend Deanne took her son for the exact same procedures: tonsil and adenoids out, ear tubes in. Like a reasonably responsible mother, Deanne followed the nurse's instructions and gave him codeine. He proceeded to throw up for five straight days. Deanne called me. "He has lost so much weight that I can see his ribs." They had stopped giving him the medication, but his stomach wouldn't settle down.

"Oh, I wish I had thought to say something to you," I offered helplessly.

"I will never give a child that strong of medicine again."

The nurse had been emphatic that without the codeine, Kate would experience excruciating pain. Kate did fine. She never even took a second dose of children's pain relief. The person who experienced excruciating pain was Deanne's son, whose codeine-induced vomiting burned his throat raw.

Why are doctors so giddy about prescribing drugs when often the side effects are worse than the symptoms of the illness? Maybe by not taking the medicine, I will give my thyroid a chance to bounce back on its own—the human body is miraculous that way.

—*◊/◊/◊*—

DR. THORPE IS waiting for me to say whether or not I want the prescription, which would signal the end of the appointment, but I have pages of questions. "I don't feel any better after taking the antivirals. I know you said they would be questionable and that the only known treatment for mono is rest and good nutrition, but the most frustrating problem is that I cannot sleep." I explain the sirens and the jolting awake. "How can I get better when I can't get a restful night's sleep?"

Dr. Thorpe says, "Often, if an adult naps during the day, they have difficulty falling asleep at night."

I feel like a reprimanded child. "I don't usually nap in the day," I answer, even though I'm trying to understand why a person with mono shouldn't rest as much as possible. "I might lie on the couch, but even then, if I try to fall asleep, something jerks me awake. You said I needed to get over the Epstein-Barr virus to see if my thyroid could get back to normal. How can I get over the virus if I can't sleep?"

"That was before we knew about the Hashimoto's," Dr. Thorpe says.

What a jumbled pile of perplexity. "What can I do to be able to sleep?"

There is a loud silence as we face each other. I know that he caught himself before offering a prescription for sleeping pills. He knows I am not going to take the Synthroid.

We are at an impasse.

Dr. Thorpe leaves with an exasperated exhale. I leave with an appointment for a follow-up thyroid test in six weeks. On the drive home I'm not feeling happy with either Dr. Thorpe or Dr. Erdmann. Why hadn't the homeopathic testing at Dr. Erdmann's office found the Hashimoto's? I saw the blood lab results myself and I do have the anti-thyroid peroxidase antibodies or whatever they're called. Maybe Dr. Erdmann is a phony, like Aaron says.

On the other hand, that lab report was four weeks old! If Dr. Thorpe really believes I won't feel better until I take Synthroid, then why didn't he call me in a prescription four weeks ago? The inconsideration of leaving me to suffer for four weeks makes me furious.

I have no idea what to do. Hashimoto's isn't a death sentence, but it is a life sentence.

IN BED THAT night I replay the appointment for Aaron. He says, "You took a questionable antiviral that you weren't sure would help, but you won't take a thyroid medicine that will?"

"The antiviral was *temporary*. If I start the thyroid pill, I will be taking it for the rest of my life. I want to give my thyroid a chance to heal on its own."

Aaron rolls away from me.

"Goodnight?" I whisper. It's all so befuddling. I thought Dr. Erdmann was my answer. It felt like God guided me to find him. Everything he said felt right. But obviously Dr. Thorpe and Aaron think he is a nutcase selling snake oil tonic.

CHAPTER 37

You Will Get 100% Well

TODAY IS TANNER'S third birthday and he has been running around all morning wearing nothing but his birthday suit. He is potty training and you could say we are using the naked technique. (Annice refers to my house as "clothing optional.") Aaron and I hand Tanner a wrapped gift. His eyes light up when he rips off the paper and finds a new rubber bat and ball. Tanner runs into our bedroom and returns wearing one of Aaron's brown belts and a ball cap. That is all he is wearing—the belt and the hat—as he proceeds to play baseball in the backyard. I try to snap a G-rated photo, but each time he takes a good hard swing, the belt falls precariously to his ankles. Aaron and I laugh behind our hands. Jack pulls himself up to standing against my patio chair.

"He's going to be walking soon," Aaron observes.

Jack's first year has gone too quickly and yet, it has been the longest year of my life.

When Tanner is down for his afternoon nap, I leave for a homeopathic treatment, unaware that it is me who is about to receive the most unexpected gift.

At my appointment I tell Dr. Erdmann about my mood swings, switching from happy as a lark to droopy as a basset hound, to angry as a bear with its paw in a hornet's nest. I'm worried he'll lock me in a looney bin, but Dr. Erdmann is casual, as if he sees this every day.

"That's your liver detoxing."

Maybe he does see it every day.

"Today we're going to do something different. Let's unbury your worries."

We do the whole muscle testing routine, only this time I'm flat on my back on the table, arm poking out like the flush handle of a toilet. Instead of poking and prodding organs, he makes a statement, then pushes down on my arm.

"You are troubled by the past."

My arm stays firmly in place.

"Your worry is in the present."

Another solid push but my arm doesn't budge.

"Your worry is in the future."

With this push my arm gives way and drops to the ground. It still freaks me out how he does that.

"Interesting," he says.

I agree. I'd like to know what worries me in the future, but Dr. Erdmann is so focused that instead of interrupting with my usual crossfire of questions, I keep quiet and let him continue.

"Your worry is about money."

My arm stays hard like a boulder, which surprises the heck out of me because I am *always* worried about money.

"You are worried about family."

My outstretched arm holds straight as a steel rod.

The questioning goes on and my arm stays firm until Dr. Erdmann says, "You are worried about health."

My arm gives out so fast under his push that Dr. Erdmann loses his balance and barely rights himself before face-planting. It takes a few minutes for us both to get our bearings.

"Now we're on to something." Dr. Erdmann plants his feet and I lift my arm out again. He rephrases the statement. "You worry that you will always be sick, that you will never get well." My arm drops like the seat of a dunking machine when the target has been hit square center. Dr. Erdmann says, "You fear that you will live with this illness for the rest of your life." With these words the table, the floor, the earth have been pulled out from under me and I am freefalling through empty space.

All of my life I have taken my body for granted. I falsely assumed I could run at any pace and my legs would always move. I expected my arms would never quit working, my brain would never stop thinking. Mine is a case of self-abuse beyond measure; so yes, what Dr. Erdmann says is true—I am afraid that I have learned my lesson too late. My punishment is justly deserved. For repeated crimes against my body, I have been sentenced to live with chronic illness.

Dr. Erdmann gets smaller as I fall away from him. The lights overhead get more distant. I am weightless in a space without gravity. My future—all my hopes and dreams—float around me, too. I'm falling for hours, maybe months, perhaps years. Time is swirling around me too, every timepiece I've ever owned—the digital dashboard clock from the Taurus, the microwave timer, the watch my parents gave me senior year of high school, my alarm clock—nothing is concrete any longer, my life has no grounding. I continue to drift, plummeting downward, but watching the dive in slow motion. There's no telling if I can regain my footing or if I will hit the bottom of the canyon floor and shatter into a million pieces.

Dr. Erdmann speaks again. His voice travels deep and catches up to my freefall. "You are afraid you won't get well, but—*my dear*—you will get one hundred percent well." His words become arms, soft yet solid arms, encircling me in a well-skilled catch, stopping my fall in the nick of time. These arms made of words lower me gently, not into a trough of icy water, but into a wooly cloud that envelops me in warmth.

Most words are heard with the ears and they sound exactly like *words*, because that's what they are. Other words bypass the ears and pierce the heart. These words aren't *heard*, they are *felt*. These words don't sound like words, they sound like…*truth*.

I will get one hundred percent well. I know it in the deepest part of me. I never have to question again.

Dr. Erdmann holds out his hand for me to grab on to and pulls me into a seated position, as he does at the end of every appointment. I reach for my shoes.

"One last thing." Dr. Erdmann is checking his notes in my file. "Do you find that you jerk awake when you're trying to fall asleep?"

My shoes hit the floor and my chin nearly does as well. "How did you know?"

"Some people say it's like they've heard an alarm."

"That is exactly what happens. I can't remember the last time I was able to fall asleep without jerking awake a half-dozen times first."

"I'm shocked how low your cortisol levels are." He points to the number sixteen on my lab reports. "Cortisol is produced in your adrenal glands. For so long your body has had to produce spurts of cortisol in order to keep you going, so now, as soon as you start to fall asleep, your body releases a surge of cortisol giving you an adrenaline rush. Then you can't fall back to sleep because you're hyped up on adrenaline. The next day, you probably want to crash—just like any person does after having an adrenalized experience. We'll get your cortisol levels regulated and you'll sleep better than a baby."

While Dr. Thorpe had rolled his eyes at my sleeping dilemma, Dr. Erdmann described word for word what I experience every night.

At the checkout counter, Julia asks, "How did it go today?" She's not making small talk. Our eyes connect and there is a brief, but real exchange of mutual connection. She knows me because she has been on my side of the counter. I wonder how she came to work with Dr. Erdmann.

"I can't describe it," I say.

She nods knowingly. "The appointment is forty-five dollars and the pro-cortisol supplement is fifteen dollars." She prints a receipt.

"Do you accept checks?"

Laiah has closed her magazine and joins me at the counter looking over my shoulder as I write the check. She's not stupid. She can do math, and she knows these appointments are adding up. Sixty dollars twice per week can buy a lot of groceries. She leans on the counter with a grim expression. "Just thinking what Aaron will say about you bringing home yet another non-FDA approved supplement," she says.

I turn away from Laiah and sign my name at the bottom of my check. *Maleah Warner.* It looks like the Jane Hancock on my personal declaration of independence. What does this sixty-dollar check declare? That I am worth the money.

I'm going to be able to sleep. I will get one hundred percent well.

Rather than carrying the weight of a life sentence of drug dependency, the pro-cortisol supplements feels light, like a little bottle of helium. By the third night on the supplement I fall asleep at the same time as Aaron. In the morning I roll toward him. "Did Jack wake up in the night?"

"I didn't hear him." Aaron looks at me. "Did you get up with him?"

"No. I slept all night."

⸺⊰⊱⸺

WE ARE GETTING everything ready to close up our house and spend two months of summer in Utah and Idaho. We've finished the June issue, forwarded our mail to my parents' address, and we have been eating through our freezer and refrigerator. There are two final missions to cross off my list before leaving town.

One is to have a final treatment with Dr. Erdmann.

"So, you're going to be gone for two months?" Dr. Erdmann asks in amazement as he presses into my back. "I guess that officially makes you snowbirds, though you're a bit young."

"Aaron's youngest brother is getting married in June and we have a family reunion in Yellowstone at the end of July, so we decided to stay the whole summer."

I've had this same conversation with so many people over the past few weeks that my answers are practically scripted. Most people reply by saying how lucky we are, which is exactly how Dr. Erdmann responds. "You're lucky. Not many people get to do that."

I suppose that by starting the magazine, we've created a certain amount of destiny for ourselves, but of all people, I would have expected Dr. Erdmann to be more perceptive about the cost of this "luck."

Dr. Erdmann pulls the bones at the base of my skull. "It's important that you continue treatments while you're gone so you don't lose the progress you've made." Dr. Erdmann gives me the contact information for one of his colleagues in Utah.

I don't want to fall backward, either, but honestly, it's hard to imagine what could be more medicinal than a summer out of the stifling heat. Unlike last summer, this year I'm not recovering from an episiotomy, and I'm not waking up in the night to breastfeed a newborn. Spending six weeks in the cool mountain air of Utah and Idaho—what could be more therapeutic? Still, I fully intend to give his colleague a call.

THE LAST THING we do before leaving town is attend a graduation. This I do with pleasure. Kate is not my first kindergarten graduate, but hers is my first kindergarten graduation. Last year Danny was so elated with his new baby brother that my absence from his kindergarten graduation didn't bother him an ounce, but it bothers me that I will never see my oldest son graduate from kindergarten. I will, however, see Kate graduate.

The school auditorium is covered with handmade decorations— colorful flowers cut and painted from rolls of school paper, children's handprints, and twisted streamers marking the aisles. The mini-sized graduates with their cardboard caps and garbage sack robes sing their songs with gusto, though slightly off-key. I'd like to petition that graduation ceremonies for anyone over the age of five be banned unless the speakers can prove as entertaining as children grabbing a microphone and boldly declaring, "When I grow up, I want to be a garbage man."

At the end of the program, Jack steps into the aisle and wobbles on unsteady legs to greet Kate. Aaron bends down to give her a flower; she throws her arms around his neck and they hug each other tight. In the post-graduation photos, my smile is not forced.

Hopefully, the worst is behind me now.

CHAPTER 38

Elevator

AS EXCITED AS I am for this summer of adventure, I'm plagued with worry that I will have a "freak-out" episode around my extended family. Other than Annice and Paul, I haven't talked with my siblings about my "condition" and I have no idea if they talk to each other about me. Will they have conversations about me when I'm not in the room? Will they grill Aaron about what's going on?

Aaron: "The doctor wanted her to start medication three months ago, but she refuses."

Family member: "Is she still going to the witch doctor?"

Aaron: "She insists it's making her better, but I don't see any difference."

Family member: "Should we check her into a psychiatric unit?"

Although I believe the treatments are working, all the detoxing and spinal adjusting and muscle testing has me feeling stripped bare. My once-strong facades are broken down and I don't like the idea of being paraded in front of family naked and exposed like a plucked chicken. I'd prefer to be alone while my liver detoxifies, my kidneys reboot, and my adrenals recharge. And even though I'm not a spokesperson for holistic medicine, the burden of proof is on me to affirm that I'm right in not taking prescription drugs.

We arrive at the cabin west of Yellowstone and the kids quickly run out to find their cousins and claim rooms with bunk beds so they can stay awake talking. Aaron hauls in suitcases while I unload groceries into the pantry and refrigerator. For the first few days, the trip goes well. Mrs. Hyde doesn't appear. I don't freak out, burst into a fit of crying, or drip emotional goo over anyone. I'm extremely cautious. At night I go to bed at the same time as the children. From my cabin room I can hear the laughter of my siblings playing games and telling jokes. I'm missing out on the fun, but I want my body to recover its natural sleep cycles and not become dependent on the pro-cortisol. In the afternoons after lunch, when everyone is draped out on couches for a midday nap, I hear Dr. Thorpe's voice in my head: "Adults who nap during the day often have trouble falling asleep at night." It's too risky to mess with my newly recovered nighttime sleep, so instead of napping, I strap the camera over my shoulder and go for a walk.

This is where it starts.

The *feeling*.

As I walk a narrow trail through aspen and pine trees, the nerves down my back shiver and my skin prickles—a "goose walked over my grave" sensation. To my left a twig snaps, and holding the camera tight like a tucked football, I run full-speed back down the trail, not stopping until I reach our cabin.

This happens the next three days. Once when I'm sitting on a bridge, my bare feet dangling in the water, I sense that someone is watching. Jumping to my feet, I look all around. It could have been a bear or a cougar. It could have been a murderer, hiding in the thick brush waiting for an unsuspecting victim. Another time I've taken a book to sit on a log bench beneath a shady tree when an ominous awareness tells me I must move, and quick! Barely gathering my book and jacket, I roll off the log and scramble several feet forward on hands and knees before working up to a run. Only after covering several yards do I turn to see if the tree fell and crushed the log. It hadn't. The scene of the log bench highlighted with a sliver of mountain sunlight through the pines is picturesque and peaceful, but my heart pounds with the urgency of trying to escape a burning building trapped by a locked door.

When I call and tell Laiah, she says, "What if it's not a feeling, what if it's a premonition?"

I don't want to believe her, but what other explanation is there? I'm staying in a beautiful cabin, nestled in a magnificent forest, surrounded by giggling children, good food, and my favorite people in all the world, and yet I cannot shake the feeling that this will be my last summer with my family. And it's not this sickness that will be the death of me. No, rather it's going to be an accident, an animal mauling, a kidnapping, a murder. This awareness doesn't settle well with me. Should I be thankful that God is cluing me in so that I can make the most of the little time I have left, or angry that His warning is making me so jittery I can't enjoy anything? Despite going to bed early, I don't sleep well at night, thinking through the numerous ways I could die here, in addition to the possibility that Aaron and the kids might be better off without me.

As sad as I am about the prospect of dying, what worries me most is that my family will mistakenly assume that I caused my own death, because *it* is on my record.

She took her own life.

She committed suicide.

They have to know I would never…but then Laiah mentions that maybe they know about the elevator incident. So when I hear the rustle in the trees behind me, once again I take off in a sprint, not stopping until I have opened the basement door of the cabin and run inside, leaning against the wall to catch my breath after locking the door behind me.

Because *depression* is in my medical records, my fear is that if anything mysterious ever happens to me, the police will immediately claim suicide, and what if my family believes them?

Especially after what happened in the elevator.

—◦◦◦—

MY PARENTS LIVE on the second floor of their Salt Lake condo building, but every time we visit, Danny and Kate insist on riding the elevator. They hit the numbers for various levels and we usually stop on every floor on our way to the top—just for kicks and giggles—before riding back down to the second floor.

When we arrived in Utah over a month ago, we drove directly to my parents' building. Aaron's youngest brother, Robert, was getting married in a few days and the wedding luncheon would be in the social room of my parents' building, since they live so close to the Salt Lake Temple where the wedding would take place. My one job for wedding preparation was to count if there was enough seating for the guests, or if the caterers needed to bring more chairs. We pulled into their parking garage on June 8, Jack's first birthday.

My mother opened the door wearing an apron; the aroma of fresh baking wafted into the hallway. "Hello guys!" She held out her arms and the kids surrounded her legs with hugs. "Come here sweet boy." She lifted Jack from my arms. "Happy birthday! Grandma has a present for you." We followed her inside.

"Yum, it smells like cake." Danny sniffed the air while Kate and Tanner ran immediately to the secret spot behind the couch where Grandma keeps her toy bucket. In no time, the bucket was emptied, every toy spread across the front room.

After dinner, Mom put one candle in a piece of cake for Jack. I held his hands down while we sang "Happy Birthday," then Danny, Kate, and Tanner helped him blow out the candle. One year ago Jack was born, one year ago Danny graduated from kindergarten. One year felt like an aeon.

Aaron had brought in our luggage from the van and I had brought in a horrible sensation of skin crawling that I couldn't shake, despite my mom's homemade dinner and the birthday fun. Helping wash dinner dishes, my heart was picking up speed, reminding me of when the kids play with the wind-up metronome on my piano. Whenever they force the metronome gauge to its lowest point until the pendulum clicks wildly back and forth, over two hundred beats per minute, I shout at them, "That's not a toy! You're going to break it." This is what my heart was doing. Clicking faster and faster until it seemed my chest would explode.

Keeping my head down and my hands in sudsy water, I scrubbed the pots and nodded while Mom updated me with news of aunts, uncles, and cousins. After dishes, Mom and I sat on the couch watching Jack push his new circus train across the carpet. Aaron, Danny, Kate, and Tanner had gone out to the balcony and were rocking on the porch swing, waving to the pedestrians strolling through Brigham Young Historic Park.

My mother's mouth moved and words swirled around my head, reporting the due dates of pregnant cousins. Then the words morphed into a buzzing and Jack's train appeared as a smear of psychedelic colors. The metronome in my chest morphed into the countdown of an explosive device. The condo walls closed in. My skin itched and I looked around to see if spiders and scorpions were pouring in through cracks in the doors and windows. Centipedes crawled up my back while I knelt down, changing Jack's stinky diaper. And somehow, I kept all these threats safely hidden from my mother. My only choice was escape.

"I'm going to throw out Jack's diaper," I called behind me, rushing to the door.

Down the hall I pounded the elevator button over and over, and continually looked up and down the hallway to see who was chasing me. Just in time the steel doors slid open and swallowed me inside the protection of its small space. My hands squeezed my head in a vice grip—a futile endeavor to push the explosion back down into the souls of my feet. The doors started to open—had my mom come looking for me? The numbers were blurry, so my hand slid down the panel, setting multiple circles aglow. Each time the elevator stopped and the doors attempted to open, I hit the *close* button with the urgent need to shut out the light of a new hallway on a new apartment level. Finally, at the thirteenth floor (marked *P* for Penthouse), my thumb held the *close* button and my forehead landed against the wall with a *thunk*. On the other side of the metal doors was a staircase to the roof, and though I'd never before set foot on the roof of my parents' building, in my mind I could see and experience every minute detail from the way the tips of my shoes looked hanging over the ledge, to how the wind felt fresh as it brushed the hair off the back of my neck.

The city skyline surrounded me in all directions: the Salt Lake Temple, the State Capitol, the East Mountains, the Western Salt Flats. Four years earlier the world had watched the Winter Olympics hosted by Salt Lake City. From our Arizona living room, we had cheered when the television camera showed this very apartment building in the background. At that time I could have never predicted imagining how it would feel to fall thirteen stories to the sidewalk below.

Would my death devastate my parents? I'd never seen my mom or dad anything but rock solid. Would this shake them—the death of their middle daughter? When an officer knocked on their apartment door, would they take his word, or would they have to see for themselves, the broken form of their girl outlined in chalk on the very path they walk every Sunday on their way to church? What would their congregation say when they heard how Howard and Maureen's adult daughter killed herself by jumping off the roof of their building, her body in pieces directly below their window? Would my death unravel them, or would they square their jaws and continue forward in their stalwart, stoic manner? My mom would cry for a few days. My dad would plan his talk for my funeral. But they would not break.

Where did I come from, then, that I break so easily?

A solid, whiny beep rang through the elevator. The doors were angry, protesting my thumb for holding them closed. I lifted my neck, feeling the blood rush to the spot where my forehead was flattened against the elevator wall. An un-sturdy step back and the bleary panel of numbers spun in a circle, seeming to lift off the panel and float in the air around me. Confused about where I was and if the pictures in my head were real—they felt so real—my fingers groped to find number two.

The elevator descent was a long exhale.

When the doors deposited me on level two, I expected to be met by a mob of people gathered with torches and pitch forks to condemn me for my treasonous phantasy. But the hall was empty.

Back inside the condo, I held Jack's innocence away from my tarnished heart.

The next day at Robert's wedding reception, images from the elevator stalked me, popping out at inopportune moments no matter the maneuvers I made to lose them. During the luncheon I boxed myself away in the kitchen, washing my hands often, not wanting a smear of my darkness spreading to the guests.

—⟋⟍⟋⟍—

THERE IS NO way anyone could possibly know about my haunted vision in the elevator. I have not breathed a word. But in any case, after locking the basement cabin door behind me, I find my journal and fill three handwritten pages of assurance that I am happy and would never—*never*—voluntarily end my life. Then I leave the notebook in a place my family can find.

On our last night in Yellowstone, Paul and I are sitting by a campfire helping the younger cousins transfer their roasted marshmallows onto graham crackers. Licking gooey marshmallow from my fingertips, I ask Paul how high my TSH number can get before I need to panic. He's not a fan of homeopathic medicine, but he's not big on drugs either, so he has no problem with me holding off on taking Synthroid. Paul has been supportive and answered all my questions the multiple times I've called him on the phone. He's seen people with a TSH of twenty-seven who didn't know they were sick, so my level six doesn't worry him. Paul grabs Tanner's roasting stick in the nick of time before the pointy end gauges Sammy's eyes. Then—out of the blue and looking straight into the fire—Paul says, "What if it's depression?"

His comment is surprising because I've never told Paul about postpartum depression or my doctor prescribing antidepressants. My parents don't know that part either.

"I don't feel depressed." I describe for Paul my image of depression as a person who stays in bed all day, not wanting to do anything, having no ambition, no goals, no desire to participate in life. "I don't feel like that at all. I care about life. I want back in the game." I pause and stir the flames with a piece of wood. "Is that depression?"

Paul tosses another log into the fire, stirring sparks that rise upward, some flicker out early, some seem to last indefinitely.

"Is it?" I ask again. "Is that depression?"

"I don't know," he says finally.

CHAPTER 39

Hurricane

IT IS THE last day of August and I'm parked outside a pharmacy drive-through where I've passed the paper prescription for Synthroid that Dr. Thorpe printed six months ago through the metal fold-out drawer and instructed the pharmacist to fill it with the generic brand.

"That'll be ready in twenty minutes," the voice crackles over the intercom.

For twenty minutes I drive the more secluded roads of Sun City Grand, fuming over how Dr. Erdmann was a bogus fake all along. Had I wanted health so desperately that I'd fabricated a false belief in his promise of getting one hundred percent well?

Back at the drive-through window, the pharmacy technician places a white paper bag in the drawer. "Take the pill at the same time every day on an empty stomach. Morning is best, about a half hour before eating breakfast. Your total is seven dollars."

Six months of spine cracking, acupuncture, arm dropping, disgusting foot baths, and $1,000, only to be right back to what Dr. Thorpe prescribed in the first place, and only seven dollars poorer. Maybe it's my fault for taking a two-month break from treatments.

AT THE END of July, we made our second return to earth's atmosphere after a summer of snowbirding. Once again, the re-acclimation to regular life had been choppy. For one, the Jack we unbuckled from the forward-facing car seat at the end of the summer was a different Jack from the barely-walking baby we'd buckled into his rear-facing car seat at the beginning of June. Where and when he learned to climb, I can't say, but now that we're home, he's constantly laddering himself onto the table, the kitchen island, even the top of the refrigerator. He's discovering new heights of exploratory opportunities that didn't exist when he was a belly crawler.

Aaron started calling him *"Hurricane"* due to his general speed, force of destruction, and the difficulty of predicting the shore on which his chaos would land. Add the fact that he drools like a Saint Bernard, and you get a combination of wind and moisture reminiscent of chasing the Tasmanian devil out of the shower. One evening I found Jack fully clothed and standing, proud as a peacock, *in* the toilet bowl, the full roll of toilet paper unwound in white layers around him. The scene brought to mind a sign that hung in the community pool of my hometown. In bold, red letters the sign read: *We don't swim in your toilet, so don't pee in our pool.* Lifting him cautiously under the arms from the porcelain basin, I could only hope the last person who used this "pool" before Jack had remembered to flush.

AT MY POST-SUMMER follow-up, Dr Thorpe said my thyroid hormone level was in the normal range, but on the high end of normal. He recommended Synthroid—again—and asked if I wanted a new prescription. I told him I still had the first prescription he gave me. At home when Aaron asked about my test results, I slapped the lab copy on the counter. He looked at the paper. "Don't you think it's time to stop ignoring the tests and take the medication?"

Standing in the kitchen with Aaron's gaze burrowing into me, an image came to mind. The end of last summer, right after we'd come home from Utah, Aaron had chaperoned a youth wilderness trek. Jack was eight weeks old or perhaps I would have tagged along. The first night at camp, a monsoon storm blew in with a ferocity that lifted ten-gallon water barrels off the ground. Shouting at each other through glassy sheets of ice-cold water, Aaron and the other men tried to call out questions and instructions to keep the teens safe, but they couldn't hear a thing—the wind drowned all communication, even when they were practically face to face.

This is what I tried to explain to Aaron, the sense that I was in the middle of a storm and people were screaming instructions at me. My body was trying to tell me something; I knew it was, but for all the noise, I couldn't understand what it was saying. I told Aaron I wasn't ignoring the tests, I was trying to discern the message. In all the commotion, I couldn't deny my gut instinct telling me this thyroid malfunction was the tip of the iceberg to deeper issues. If taking Synthroid helped to ease my symptoms, would I pull back into the fast lane of life and stop looking for answers? "I'm trying to heal *completely*," I told him. "I don't want a Band-Aid fix. I want to get to the core problem."

"That doesn't make any sense." His voice raised with intensity. "You are destroying your body."

That night I thrashed around in bed. My pro-cortisol pills were gone, and I refused to get more because the point of homeopathic treatment was to *not* take pills for the rest of my life. Listening to Aaron snore peacefully, I wanted to put a cinderblock in my pillow and knock him in the face. Instead, I left to wrestle out the night on the family room couch, disturbed by gruesome dreams of finding Kate dead, hanging upside down, her toenails and fingernails torn off and dripping blood.

Aaron walked out in the early dawn. "Why can't you stand to sleep by me? Do I repulse you?"

Despite my reassurance that this sleeping issue was all parts me and zero parts him, I could tell he didn't believe me.

FULLY INTENDING TO resume treatments with Dr. Erdmann, I returned to his office a few days after the appointment with Dr. Thorpe. He greeted me with his jolly "Hey! How are ya? How was your summer?" While repeating muscle testing and making adjustments to my spine, Dr. Erdmann proceeded to describe a new treatment regimen. With an abundance of exuberance, he explained the background of an allergy-reduction program and shared the testimonial of a client who was so allergic to carrots she couldn't be within one hundred feet of a carrot without having an allergic reaction. Then, after finishing this particular treatment, she became popular in her neighborhood for baking the most delectable carrot cake. I'd never heard of anyone being allergic to carrots.

Unlike my first meeting with Dr. Erdmann, nothing about this regimen felt right to me. Instead of standing up and voting in unanimous favor, my cells were pleading, *Please don't put us through another six months of this. We've been fighting so long, we don't have strength for another battle.*

"I can't start a new round of treatments." I told him. "I have tried, but I'm not getting any better. My body can't take any more."

Dr. Erdmann would have been justified bringing up the fact that I didn't see his colleague in Utah—not one time—over the summer, but instead he surprised me by saying, "I think you're right. Sometimes your body needs outside support while it's working on healing." He suggested that I take a "natural" thyroid supplement which does basically the same thing as Synthroid, but is derived "naturally" from the thyroids of pigs or cows instead of being synthetically created in a lab.

My mind drew a cartoon image of me swallowing the pills and slowly growing a snout and a curly pink tail. "Will it make me oink?"

Dr. Erdmann laughed, but I wasn't amused. How "natural" is ingesting swine hormones?

I went home and mulled over the options for a few days, did some research, then returned to Dr. Erdmann's office. "I need to stop treatment." I gave him a spiel that sounded a lot like I was breaking up with a boyfriend: It's not you, it's me. I need a break. My body needs a break. My bank account needs a break. I thanked him for all his help. He told me to come back as soon as I was ready to resume.

At the last minute a question popped out of my mouth—no idea where it came from. "Can you recommend any books that might help me?"

He nodded and wrote a title on the top of my notebook page. "Call my office anytime." Dr. Erdmann patted my shoulder. I had no doubt he was being sincere.

I paid for the visit by debit card and shook my head when Julia asked if I wanted to schedule another appointment. In my car I pounded the steering wheel and screamed. The whole drive to the pharmacy I teetered about whether my treatments with Dr. Erdmann had done any good or if they'd all been a well-played con. What about how he'd found a buildup of thallium in my body though I'd never told him about growing up near coal-burning power plants? And the foamy mucus in the water around my feet when I'd been coughing up phlegm for months? And the adrenal burnout…everything he said had made so much sense to me, but in the end he'd offered the same—albeit "natural"—drug as Dr. Thorpe.

<hr />

WITH THE WHITE paper prescription bag sitting on the passenger seat, I stop at the library to check out the book Dr. Erdmann recommended. It isn't in their collection, but the clerk helps me fill out a request for interlibrary loan.

At home I open the front door to find Jack seated nobly atop the piano in the spot reserved for the bust of Chopin. He is pounding keys with his feet and shaking clouds of baby powder onto stacks of music books scattered over the floor. A trail of drool has drawn tracks in the dust on the piano, so one might think a snail crawled across the lid. "Come here, Pal." I hoist him onto my hip and wipe his mouth dry with my sleeve. "You are a hurricane."

CHAPTER 40

Body Worlds

DANNY WAS ABOUT five years old when he came to me one day with a ringing in his ears. He'd never experienced ear-ringing before and struggled finding words to describe it. He told me he had a sound in his ears and explained it this way: "I think God is talking," he said, cupping his hands over both ears, "but I don't know what He's trying to say."

Me too, Danny. What does it mean, this noise and disruption, this ringing in my ears? Recently I read that pain and sickness are the body's way of sounding a warning bell to call attention to the fact that the spirit is diseased. Is that what I'm hearing? A warning bell?

For a year I've been pleading for God to make me well again. Teaching the New Testament, I became familiar with the stories of Jesus' miraculous healings. He rubbed dirt into a blind man's eyes and the man could see again. Jaurius' daughter was dead and Jesus called her back to life. The woman who spent all her money on doctors—she and I could be pen pals, except her story had a seemingly simple ending. She touched the bottom of Jesus's robe and was healed. My story is still going.

I'm intrigued how healing takes place in different ways for different people. Some are healed outright by merely asking. Some are required to take action, like dipping seven times in a river. Some are carried to their miracle by the faith of others. Sometimes people had to be in Jesus' presence while others were healed long distance.

What about me? Do I need to bathe in the River Jordan? Do I need a troupe of friends to lower me through a thatched roof?

The theme for the women's church social this month is Indonesian Cultural Night. Seeing as how transporting my body from home to any other location nearly requires a forklift and industrial straps, I almost don't go, but miraculous things tend to happen when women gather, and I am in the market for a miracle. The speaker mentions little about her Indonesian culture and mostly relates the story of being abandoned by her husband and left to provide for her children alone. She said, "For a long time I questioned God, 'Why me?' then I changed my prayer to 'Help me' and after that everything transformed." She found a job, raised her kids, and became stronger than she knew she could be.

Back at home I change my prayer from *heal me* to *help me. What does my body need me to know?* Rather than begging God to take *it* away, to make *it* all better, I start saying, "Teach me about *it.*"

I think there's an old adage about how if a student shows up hungry for answers, a teacher will appear with a combo meal. Teachers show up for me in a variety of shapes, forms, and guises—some of them plastic.

It's a Friday night and Aaron and I go on a date to the Arizona Science Center to tour Gunther Von Hagens' *Body Worlds*. On exhibit are real human bodies preserved through a process of plastination. The bodies are posed in various forms of human experience: catching a ball, riding a horse, ice skating. According to exhibit literature, the bodies were donated to Von Hagen's institute by the people who lived in the bodies prior to their natural deaths and with full knowledge of being preserved and studied for years beyond death by having their internal liquids replaced with plastic upon their departure. None of the exhibits have skin, so their former identity is unrecognizable. Where these "people" who once inhabited these bodies are now is a debate that has inflamed science and religion for centuries. Without getting entangled in that debate, I will simply add my own humble opinion that—as I stare at molded faces, hardened torsos, statue-like arms and legs—those "people" are not *here*.

The miracle of Von Hagen's plastination is that every microscopic detail of the human physique can be preserved in exquisite detail without decay, discoloration, or smell of formaldehyde. I spend ten solid minutes staring at the perfectly preserved circulatory system of a human face. Every vein, every artery that pumped blood to the person's cheeks when blushing is here for me to examine. What is missing is the emotion that caused the individual to blush. What had happened? What was he or she thinking and feeling? Who was the personality around the intricate highway of blood vessels?

The piece I can't stop staring at is a body posed with arm outstretched and holding its skin loose in its hand as if it had just undressed and was going to toss the skin in the laundry basket like worn pajamas. Studying the figure, I can't tell eye color, hair color, or ethnicity. I can't judge if the face had a flawless complexion or was riddled with acne. Without skin, the "person" is all muscles, bones, and organs. There is no indication of popularity, social status, or income level. No signs of race, religion, class, or IQ. The exhibit demonstrates one thing plainly: On the inside, we really are all the same. I am transfixed. By stepping out of the skin, this person has stepped out of all stereotypes. The skin looks so heavy, like the poor arm will break under the weight.

Aaron comes back and takes my hand, urging me to move ahead. Our babysitter must be home by 10:00. Moving through the museum, we study brains, hearts, lungs, stomachs and examine every system of the human body from digestive to nervous. I see placentas encasing tiny fetuses with perfectly formed fingernails. There are kidneys, spleens, and livers. What I do not see is human individuality. None of these organs or cells or tissues are the source of personality. There is no consciousness here.

The experience at the museum does two things for me. One, it reiterates my long-held belief that *I* am not my body, and somehow this understanding makes me also understand that *I* have not been listening to my body. We are separate entities, my body and *me*, but for now *we* are symbiotically intertwined. We are interdependent, my body and *me*, and *I* have been a careless, irresponsible roommate.

All my life I've worn busyness and exhaustion as a badge of honor. Running my body into the ground has been my attempt to earn worthiness, to prove I'm the opposite of lazy. And for the past year I've been trying to force my body to snap back into being an indefatigable slave to my image of perfection. For the first time, my heart is cracked open to the idea that life could be something else.

In the slightest way, I'm beginning to see the flicker of possibility that it's possible to live without carrying the weight of flawless skin.

CHAPTER 41

Magpie

FOR SEVEN DAYS I've swallowed those little thyroid pills without noticing much difference, then today, I wake up with enough energy to leave the house and take Tanner and Jack to story time at the library. The new Surprise library, built in 2002, is state of the art compared to the old one-room house where I used to take Danny and Kate faithfully every week. This library is closer with quadruple the collection, but I've never brought Tanner and Jack to story time here. My ulterior motive for the outing is to pick up my library loan book before it gets returned to its home library tomorrow. Under the W's, I see my name poking out from a book entitled *Change Your Brain, Change Your Life*. I'm embarrassed the subtitle is exposed for all to see: *The Breakthrough Program for Conquering Anxiety, Depression, Obsessiveness, Anger, and Impulsiveness*. An acquaintance has a book on hold next to mine, and I wonder how many people have seen my name attached to this book about depression.

Later, after lunch, the boys go down for naps, Aaron heads to Goodyear, and with no piano students arriving, there is a rare pocket of solitude about the house. Gathering the book along with a journal and pencil, I go to my bedroom and settle in the rocking chair to study.

Interesting. The author's last name is Amen, like the final word of a prayer.

The introduction explains that if I'm anxious, depressed, prone to anger, or easily distracted, I might worry the problem is "all in my head." (How did he know?) Dr. Amen's research in brain scans has shown that many perceived *psychological* issues are actually problems with the *physiology* of the brain. He has my rapt attention. Is it possible my struggles arise from something physically broken in my brain, and not because I'm weak?

My cardinal rule is to read books from cover to cover starting with page one and continuing to the end, never jumping ahead to see how the story ends. This time I find the table of contents and skip directly to the chapter my body tells me I need: *The Limbic System.* Page thirty-seven informs me that an overactive limbic system causes decreased motivation and difficulty getting out of bed and moving through the day. *(Really?)* Furthermore, a malfunctioning limbic system results in appetite and sleep problems *(No way!)*, seeing life events as negative, and experiencing floods of negative emotions. *(He's describing my life to the letter.)*

With pen and notebook ready, I can hardly wait to dig into chapter four, the prescription for deep limbic healing, when a door slams and Laiah's voice calls hello.

"What are you up to?" She enters carrying her clipboard, as usual, and perches on the armrest of the loveseat.

"I just put the boys down for naps." I whisper, hoping she'll get the hint. "And I'm going to read this book that has been collecting dust on the library loan shelf for two weeks."

"Really?" Laiah cocks an eyebrow. "Reading?"

"I know. You don't have to say it. There are a million things that need to get done." Lunch dishes are still on the table. Kate's broken sandal needs to be glued.

"Okay, then. Don't mind me." Laiah folds her legs, cocks her chin, and studies the clipboard.

I proceed to read: *To heal deep limbic system problems, we need to focus on accurate thinking, the proper management of memories...*

"When do you expect Aaron back?" Laiah's question makes me automatically check the time on the clock. "Doesn't Aaron regard reading as a waste of time, especially if there's work to be done?"

What if Aaron walked in right now and saw me reading? My heartbeat takes on a level of panic. *He would think me a lazy faker, playing sick so I could get out of working in Goodyear to stay home and read.*

"A man should never find his wife being idle." Laiah scratches a note on her clipboard.

Closing Dr. Amen's book, I jump to my feet and flit around. *I have to look busy when Aaron comes in.* What to do? I need something visible like vacuum lines in the carpet or something baking in the oven. He has to be able to *see* what I've accomplished.

My feet are primed to sprint from the starting gate when I hear the voice of the woman from Indonesian Cultural Night.

Help me. Teach me.

Recently, I heard a speaker say that the only thing we really need to do every day is to feel the love of God. In the New Testament there is a story about Mary and Martha hosting Jesus for dinner. Whenever our church missionaries come for dinner, I pull out all the stops, baking homemade rolls, brownies, and sauce from scratch. I can't imagine the prospect of cooking for Jesus. When he arrives, Martha is running around, stirring the gravy so it doesn't get lumps, and setting place mats and matching dinnerware from Ikea. (The story goes something like that, it's been a year since I read it.) Meanwhile, Mary welcomes Jesus, tells him to make himself comfortable in the front room, then *sits* at his feet listening to his stories. All fired up with vexation, Martha stomps into the front room and tattles to Jesus that Mary isn't helping. Calmly Jesus says, "Martha, you're fantastic. Dinner smells delicious. Mary needs one thing tonight. Will you give us a minute, please?" (I might be paraphrasing.) After dinner, Mary cleans up all the dishes and Martha gets her time with Jesus. (At least, that's how I think it ends.)

One thing is needful. Help me. Teach me.

So instead of mixing dough for a homemade pie, I pick up Dr. Amen's book again and head for the family room. A beautiful October day has settled around our house. The summer heat is gone and Aaron has removed the dark sunscreens from the windows. Before sitting in a new study spot in the comfy corner of our sectional, I pull open the drapes, allowing unfiltered light to pour onto my face and fill the room. Settling into the sunniest spot of the couch, I reopen the book to pages showing images of healthy limbic systems compared to overactive limbic systems. Dr. Amen explains that people with limbic glitches are bombarded by a continuous replay of hopeless, dispiriting thoughts. This brain malfunction causes people to suffer from what Dr. Amen calls *ANTs* or *automatic negative thoughts*. These ANTs are an unrelenting army which volley machine gun fire in the form of hopeless phrases such as: "I should have done much better. I'm a failure. No one appreciates me." As a result, people with this condition feel regret about the past, anxiety about the future, and dissatisfaction in the present.

These people sound like me.

What he explains next makes me feel like I've made a major breakthrough in molecular theory.

Thoughts are real.

What?!

A thought is an electric signal sent through the brain. Thoughts are as real and as powerful as electricity. My hand moves quickly across the paper, taking notes and highlighting text. I am absorbing every word and concept until... Laiah enters making a ruckus in the kitchen, scooping dirty dishes, clanging them in the sink along with the ones from breakfast. Opening the dishwasher to unload the clean dishes, she gives me a look that says, *You should be doing this*, and glances at the clock to show that an hour has already passed. My afternoon is nearly gone, and I haven't accomplished anything. I stand to go do the dishes.

One thing is needful.

Taking Dr. Amen and my notebook, I open the door to the back patio and shut Laiah inside. It's the most lovely, room temperature weather. Overhead the sky is blue with puffs of cotton-white clouds. My eyes close letting the sun glow on my face. Stretching my legs out on the grass, I reopen the book and follow Dr. Amen's instruction on how to exterminate ANTs.

Write them down.

On a fresh, blank page of notebook, my pencil presses, poised and ready, but nothing comes out of its pointed graphite tip.

What are my ANTs? Do I have an ANT problem, as Dr. Amen suggests all people do? What automatic negative thoughts repeat over and over in my mind like a broken record?

Suddenly the pencil is flying across the page.

My Automatic Negative Thoughts:

ANT 1: My husband doesn't love me.

ANT 2: After years of marriage, my husband has discovered that his initial high impression of me was inaccurate. He is disappointed with me and wishes I were a more capable person.

ANT 3: My husband quantifies my time. He thinks I should use my time differently than I do.

ANT 4: By having and taking care of children, I have given up my chance to achieve significant success in my life.

ANT 5: The person whose name is on the paycheck has superiority over the person who cares for the home and kids.

ANT 6: Aaron never notices the good things I do.

When at last the pencil stops scribbling, I lift my hand from the paper, stretching it open and shut against the cramps, then shake off the pins and needles sensation that comes after having written fast and hard. I flip the page back and forth, astonished that I've filled two sheets with pencil markings, but they seem to be nothing more than pages of scribbles. Then, on closer examination, individual letters appear before my eyes, and each individual alphabet letter joins with other letters to make words. The words join together to make...sentences. These sentences, repeated over and over constitute my...*thoughts*.

ANT 7: *Being a mother isn't enough.*

ANT 8: *Nothing I do is ever enough.*

ANT 9: *I'm not enough.*

My paper goes dark. In the shadow, the curved shapes of letters linked together across the page seems to create an image. I hold the paper out in front of my face, tilting and turning, angling the paper toward the light, trying to see the hidden image. My hand had written so fast, pushing heavy on the pencil forming letters thick and bold. In my untidy cursive, the letters appear shackled together, as if handcuffed to their neighbor by heavy-laden graphite.

Chains.

Line after notebook line is filled with lengths of chain. I have been prisoner to these words for years, but somehow the process of writing out these thoughts has unlocked their hold on me. The words look weak and powerless dressed in number two-point graphite, crouching in uneven huddles on the lined paper of a ten-cent notebook.

Where had these ANTs come from? Who introduced such ignoble notions into my personal space? Did I begin life with these sentiments as an innocent baby? Surely not. Then who first spoke these words in my mind? And worse, who has repeated them over and over like an old, broken record player?

A black silhouette casts a shadow over the page. Following the shadow across the grass, I look up and find the source of the dark. Laiah is perched in our palm tree. She looks so out of place sitting in a tree while dressed in a black and white business suit. She tilts and turns her head, looking everywhere but at me. With the sun lighting her from behind, for the first time I notice her glossy eyes.

"*This* is what has plagued me for years?" I shake my notebook at her. At long last I understand what my body has been trying to tell me.

Laiah swoops down from the tree and stands between me and the paper, her figure blocking the sun. With arms crossed over her chest, she taps her foot impatiently. "Do you know how long you've been lounging out here? It's nearly 3:00 and what have you achieved today—a library trip and a few nap time books? You are always so unproductive. No wonder Aaron is constantly disappointed in you. You should be cleaning house and preparing a nice dinner to prove that you deserve his love."

Yesterday I might have fallen for Laiah's little game and dashed into the kitchen to start cooking, but now I am hearing her words, as if for the first time. And they sound a lot like the words scribbled over two pages in the notebook I'm holding. She hops nervously in a circle around me, worried about the look of revelation in my eyes. Still, she doesn't let up. "Aaron has carried all the weight of this magazine since you got sick. He's doing his job and yours, so if he comes home and has to make dinner after discovering that you've idled your afternoon in the sun, he'll regret marrying such an incompetent slouch."

In the past I would have accepted Laiah's statements at face value and allowed them to sink into my skin and settle like poison in my blood. Instead, at this moment, I *hear* Laiah's words and recognize that she is merely restating *ANT #3: My husband quantifies my time.* She's doctored up the vocabulary and personalized the specifics, but the meaning is the same as hundreds of various phrases she's harpooned at me for years: *Aaron doesn't love you.*

Focusing back on the paper and ignoring Laiah's blather, I let my hand loose to write again. This time, following Dr. Amen's instructions for exterminating *automatic negative thoughts*, I write my own response to each numbered *ANT*.

Next to *ANT #4: By having and taking care of children I have given up my chance to achieve significant success in my life,* I write:

Truth #4: Children do not detract from my life, they add to it. Being a mother is a successful occupation.

So preoccupied watching my messages of truth stream onto the paper, I don't notice them until my hand stops and I look up. Dozens of black and white magpies have landed in my yard. They squawk, making horrific noise, each one trying to outdo its neighbor. *Aaron doesn't love you. Aaron regrets marrying you. Being a mother isn't enough. Your children prevent you from being successful. You have to make money to be worthwhile.* Around me the birds swoop, hover, hop, land—just like that day with Ms. Wickersham—closing in on me, their cawing growing louder and louder until the noise is unbearable. Holding my hands over my ears, I stand up, and lengths of chain fall to the ground around my feet.

I know exactly who has repeated these toxic phrases to me. With my ears covered and my head cowered to avoid the beating of wings and beaks circling around me, I search for her.

Laiah.

She's in the middle of the thickest cluster of birds. The magpies perch on her shoulders, her head, one is eating out of her palm. She squawks at them and they answer. She pets the birds, acting nonchalant, but I see she has pecked at a hangnail on her finger until it bleeds. She strokes a magpie and pretends not to notice that I am coming toward her, but she is shaking. Our relationship—hers and mine—is about to get choppy. All the months of waiting. All the searching. I know exactly why I am sick.

"This is what has made me unhappy in my own life? This is what has weighed me down and made me feel worthless?" Laiah steps back as I thrust my notebook at her. "These weak words have made me believe that everything about my life is wrong!"

Laiah bites her lip and taps at the grass with her foot.

"And"—I pause for emphasis—"they aren't even *true!*"

Laiah keeps her head down but looks up through her bangs.

"Lai-ah." I stretch the syllables of her name. "*Laiah Papaya.*" All these years she has been my constant companion. She has been my first go-to for advice. We've been so intertwined—almost the same person—that it never occurred to me the things she says might not be *true*. In my head I hear the chime of an old schoolyard chant: *Liar, liar, pants on fire.*

Lai-ah.

Li-ar.

"You are a *liar!*"

She backs away across the gravel until she bumps into the tree. I snarl like a guard dog who has cornered a thief in the night. Laiah straightens up a little and defaults to her same old song and dance. Flapping her arms, she dances about. "Look what a sloth you've become. Come on. Get going. You could have taught four piano lessons in the amount of time you've been out here dawdling. What will Aaron think?"

Dr. Amen says to talk back to automatic negative thoughts with statements of truth. I press forward. "Aaron wants me to be happy! He wants me to use my time doing things that will make me *happy.*"

Laiah fidgets over what card to play next. "He didn't give you a gift for your birthday because he didn't think you deserved a present. You are so weak and broken that he can't even love you anymore."

Instinctively I recoil, the sting of Laiah's words landing like a swarm of mosquitos on my skin, but then I pause and *listen*. She's not saying anything clever, wise, or even accurate. She's only repeating that same old ANT #1 that Aaron doesn't love me.

Planting my feet deep in the grass, I point my finger at her nose. "Aaron loves me or he wouldn't have asked me to marry him." A flood of warmth surges through my body, breaking a dam and releasing water into my dry, brittle organs. I can physically *feel* Aaron's love. My mind floods with memories: the emotion on Aaron's face when he kissed me on our wedding day, the first Mother's Day present he gave me, that time he kicked his own client out of our house for disrespecting me. "Aaron doesn't love me because of a clean house or a homemade dinner. He loves *me* and nothing I do changes his love for me." As the words leave my mouth, I hear them for what they are: *truth.*

Speaking of truth, I must stop here with a confession. When Dr. Amen suggested writing a rational response to each automatic negative thought, I balked at the notion thinking, *This is stupid. This is nothing more than replacing a false negative with a false positive.* I had no interest in playing that old psychology game about whether the glass is half empty or half full. But speaking the words out loud, I know something that I haven't known for a very long time.

Aaron loves me.

I *know* it. And I can *feel* it. Because for the first time in a long time, I'm allowing myself to *believe* it.

Laiah pulls back her head and tries to speak, but I don't let her chirp a word. The notebook is held plain in front of her face so she can read the words: *ANT #1: Aaron doesn't love me.*

"You said this was true." I point to the statement.

She raises her hands in defense. "I never said it was true. I just said it. You decided what was true."

I drop the notebook to my side, astounded.

Laiah capitalizes on my silence. "Aaron has carried the weight of the magazine since you got sick. He's tired of doing his work and yours." Laiah can see the change in my face and she looks excited. She is antsy, waiting to see how I'll respond.

I never said it was true. I just said it. You decided what was true.

Laiah is waiting (and I get the impression she has been waiting for a long time) for *me* to tell *her* the truth. "Aaron wants me to get well. He loves *me.* More than anything else, Aaron wants me to be as healthy and as happy as I can possibly be."

The sun rises higher in the sky, reminding me that sunlight provides both warmth and visibility. My bones, which have been empty and cold for months, feel as if warm cocoa has been poured into the marrow. In my mind's eye, I see all the times Aaron came home and made dinner or cleaned the house. He wasn't saying that I should have had dinner already made or that I should be a better housekeeper. He was showing me that he *loves* me. I can't believe I've never seen it before. I want to do cartwheels across the grass. For years I've believed that Aaron detested living with me, and it has all been a *lie*. In working so hard trying to be a successful woman, I've deprived Aaron and the kids of having the woman they really want: *me*.

For the first time ever, Laiah is speechless, but I have something to say.

"Are you even real?" I ask Laiah.

"I am as real as you are," Laiah answers. "I am *you*."

"You are not *me*. I don't know who you are, but you are not *me*."

Dr. Amen recommends challenging your automatic negative thoughts and I plan to do just that. I don't know who Laiah is, but no longer will I permit her to escapade in my life unquestioned.

CHAPTER 42

Now I'm Depressed

A FEW WEEKS into taking the thyroid medication, an interesting thing happens. I begin to feel depressed. It's as if up until now my body was too far gone to even create the feeling of depression. Now that Synthroid is providing some support, my body has just enough strength to successfully be depressed.

It's great knowing *about* Laiah, but I don't know what to do *with* her. Getting rid of her would require chopping off my own head, and that's not the outcome I've been working toward. What's fascinating to me is how she's always been around and how little I've noticed her. I've always acted on her words without really hearing them.

There's a story about a traveler who discovers a village of indigenous people who live at the base of a three-hundred-foot waterfall. The scenery is picturesque, lush and green, trees laden with every sort of fruit—a literal Garden of Eden—but the sound of the waterfall is deafening, and it never stops. All day and all night as the man stays in his guest hut in this paradise, he is close to going crazy with the sound of the waterfall. One day he asks the village chief, *How do you stand the noise?* The chief replies, *What noise?* And the man says, *The noise from the waterfall.* The chief stares blankly. *What waterfall?* The villagers had grown so accustomed to the continual sound of water crashing that they didn't hear it anymore.

This happens when we no longer hear the ticking of the bedroom clock or the hum from the air conditioner.

This happened to me with Laiah. She produced such a constant dialogue in my head, that I didn't hear her. I believed anything and everything she communicated without really listening to the message.

These revelations have me teeming with questions, but rather than feeling hopeless like I did in Dr. Thorpe's office, these questions excite me.

Who is Laiah, exactly? Is she my brain? Is she my thoughts? Where do thoughts come from?

Dr. Amen says a thought is an electric signal sent through the brain. This notion that thoughts are as real and as powerful as electricity reminds me of what happened to my favorite climbing tree. Growing up, the front yard of my pink farm house was shaded by the branches and leaves of four huge trees. During a thunderstorm, the tree closest to the road was struck by lightning. The power of the lightning bolt shot through the tree and exploded a hefty piece of concrete out of our driveway. The tree itself appeared unscathed and I begged my dad not to pull it out. It looked perfectly healthy on the outside, but Dad decided the tree had to come out before a minor windstorm blew it over onto our roof. The chain on his tractor yanked out the trunk, revealing that the inside of the tree was completely black, fried all the way down to its roots.

"Lightning did that?" I said to my dad.

He answered, "Lightning is concentrated electric power. Never underestimate what electricity can do."

The volley of constant negative thoughts fired by Laiah over the years has fried my body. It's not obvious by looking at me, but my innards are torched.

Another discovery courtesy of Dr. Amen is that emotions are real and tangible in the way that liquid nitrogen is real and tangible. I used to think of emotions as ethereal concepts that existed in a floaty sphere, more adjective than substance. Anger, surprise, loathing, love. What is it that makes us *feel* emotion? Why does my heart race when I'm surprised or scared? How do butterflies of nervousness work? Why does my chest seem to swell when I see Kate learning to ride her new bike without training wheels? These are real physical reactions to emotional experiences. How does it work?

Dr. Amen says that feelings are chemicals created by thoughts. The electric pulses of thoughts trigger the brain to release chemicals into the body, and when these chemicals brush across nerve endings, we physically experience sensations known as *feelings*.

I try to think about it this way: Every color of paint offered in the Sherwin Williams catalogue is a combination of the three primary colors: red, yellow, and blue. Every emotion experienced by the human body is a combination of three main brain chemicals: dopamine, serotonin and norepinephrine. (There are more brain chemicals, but for my sake, I need to keep it simple.) The brain contains shelves full of cookbooks containing recipes for hundreds of "feelings." Like a restaurant chef slaving over a hot stove, the brain is constantly preparing dishes according to whatever the customers—*thoughts*—have ordered.

When I think a thought, I have placed an order in the Restaurant of Emotions and the chef is going to season my plate with pleasure or poison according to my demands.

No wonder I'm sick.

Once the brain has been cooking up venom soup for so long, it forgets how to make joy Jello or happiness hamburgers. For years I have simmered my organs in toxic marinade, then questioned why my systems won't function. I owe my legs, my lungs, and my liver the world's biggest apology. I wonder how I can make amends with my muscles.

Organs can malfunction. For example, a liver can become insulin-resistant or kidneys can become less efficient at filtering the blood. The brain, as an organ, can also malfunction. The brain can misfire and release recipes for emotions such as depression or anxiety into the body without being asked.

This is what I am experiencing. My body is releasing the chemical recipes for sadness, despair, worthlessness—so I am feeling these emotions, even though nothing in my life would logically trigger these emotions. If my brain is misfiring, then getting off my butt and getting to work is not going to fix it. The light is gradually dawning that I might not be able to elbow grease my way out of this.

IN THE OFFICE, the computer screen lights up. A few clicks on the keyboard and the google search bar takes me to WebMD. This is far from my first visit to this web address. In the past I've searched childhood immunizations, pinworm, fifth disease, postpartum thyroiditis, Epstein-Barr, chronic fatigue, multiple sclerosis, cancer, and Hashimoto's. Tonight, for the first time, I type in "symptoms of depression" expecting to read a list along the lines of: feeling lackluster, showing disinterest in life or relationships, lack of caring, extreme sadness, inability to cope with responsibility, desire to shut down, etc. Here is the actual list:

1. difficulty concentrating, remembering details, and making decisions
2. a foggy or muddy head
3. fatigue and decreased energy
4. feelings of guilt, worthlessness, and/or helplessness
5. feelings of hopelessness and/or pessimism
6. insomnia, early-morning wakefulness, or excessive sleeping
7. irritability, restlessness
8. loss of interest in activities or hobbies once pleasurable, including sex
9. overeating or appetite loss
10. persistent aches or pains, headaches, cramps, or digestive problems
11. persistent sad, anxious, or "empty" feelings
12. unusual preoccupation with death, accidental or intentional

Number twelve knocks the air out of my lungs. *Unusual preoccupation with death.* Is it possible my death premonitions aren't real? These horrific scenes that flash onto my mental movie screen, are they because my brain is broken? They aren't a sign from God?

My future is unveiling for me in a whole new way. Discovering Laiah for who she is has unlocked a world of possibility. It's possible that I'm *not* a failure. It's possible that I'm *not* a disappointment. It's possible that I *am loved.* Reading that one complication of depression can be an unusual preoccupation with death opens this possibility: *I'm not going to die!*

It is possible I have depression.

The website explains that having five or more symptoms is evidence of depression. I have all twelve. In a big way. This should be such a horrid revelation, but I'm so relieved by the newsflash about not dying that I clap my hands in front of my chest and collapse back against the chair with a dazed sort of satisfaction.

It's depression. I have depression!

AARON COMES WITH me to Dr. Thorpe's office. I need moral support to go through with accepting a prescription for an antidepressant. Maybe if the medicine were called a neural stimulator or proneural balancer. "Anti" sounds so rebel military faction.

This is the first time Dr. Thorpe, Aaron, and I have been in an exam room together. They graciously wait for my lead. Laiah and I rehearsed this moment extensively, but never got the wordage right. What am I supposed to say: "So I've been thinking that I might have depression, and even though I haven't wanted to take any other medication you've prescribed for me, I'd like to try some antidepressants"?

Instead, I take out my red medical notebook and read off symptoms as though I have very scientifically been studying myself and jotting down my observations—which I suppose I have. After a minute Dr. Thorpe says, "Do you have a history of depression in your family?"

"No," I say.

"Yes!" Aaron interjects.

"What do you mean?" I look at Aaron.

"She has at least two family members who have taken medication for anxiety and depression."

Dr. Thorpe and I answer at the same time. "Really?"

"How would you know that if I don't even know that?" I ask Aaron. He's never mentioned it. "Who?" I want to know. Aaron gives a look that says, *I'll tell you later.* In my family we were raised to be so good at keeping secrets.

All the reasons I don't want to take an antidepressant spill out. "I already have to take the thyroid medicine, so now will I have to take two pills every day for the rest of my life? I don't want to live dependent on drugs."

"A lot of people take an antidepressant for a period of time and then find they don't need it anymore," Dr. Thorpe offers.

"But if I have to go through a weaning phase to get myself off a drug, why don't I just go through the weaning phase now? Why can't I get my body to mend itself?"

"Sometimes the body needs to be reminded what it's supposed to do on its own. A drug can reboot your system, or you might have to take it the rest of your life. We really don't know."

"How will I know what is me and what is the pill?" I ask. "I don't want artificial love, patience, happiness, and intelligence that come from a bottle."

"What you feel right now? Is that you?" Dr. Thorpe asks.

"No, I don't feel like myself at all."

"The purpose of an antidepressant isn't to create a false you, it's to give your body support so you can be the real you."

Dr. Thorpe writes a prescription for sertraline. I don't reach out to take it, but Aaron does.

"One last question," I say. "What causes depression? Why do some people get it and some people don't?"

Dr. Thorpe closes his laptop. "Are you familiar with dogs?" I assume the statement is rhetorical. "Different breeds of dogs are known for having better temperaments than other breeds." This is going somewhere, I presume. "People are like dogs. Some have better temperaments than others."

The room is silent.

I wonder how my ancestors are responding to this valuation of our lineage. Did Dr. Thorpe just put me in the same category as an unbred pound mutt?

Bless his heart.

Driving to the pharmacy, I apologize to my pioneer forebears who possibly traveled in the same wagon train as Dr. Thorpe's progenitors. Were they forced by the Thorpe family purebreds to the back of the line for their ill temperaments? I try to focus on good thoughts and not on what Laiah is telling me that Dr. Thorpe thinks of the people for whom he prescribes *anti*depressants.

Hopefully, I won't run into anyone I know at the pharmacy. This is different from elementary school when I wanted to break my arm and get a cast for the attention. I have no intention to take my pill bottle to moms group for my friends to sign.

"That will be seventy-five dollars," the pharmaceutical technician voices through the intercom.

"Is that a ninety-day supply?"

He looks. "It's a thirty-day supply."

Seventy-five dollars? Every month? For the rest of my life? Now I really am depressed.

A FEW DAYS later we arrive at Annice's house for Thanksgiving dinner. I am quivering the way my kids do dripping wet out of the hot tub on a cold night.

"They say it takes a few weeks to adjust to medication," she tries to console me.

For sixteen days I swallow the sertraline pill. For sixteen days I'm ready to jump out of my skin. I need to explode, but I can't figure out how to explode in a socially acceptable way. The good news is that I'm sleepy. The bad news is that once I've fallen asleep, I can't wake up again. No amount of sleep is enough.

At my follow-up visit I tell Dr. Thorpe, "The sertraline is expensive. Is it possible to get a prescription for one hundred milligrams and cut the pill into five pieces to bring down the cost?"

Dr. Thorpe says, "You don't have to take sertraline. Let's change the medication. A lot of people do well with good old Prozac. It's time-tested and it's cheap."

I start with ten milligrams, the smallest possible dose. At the drive-up window the pharmacist grabs the microphone. "That will be five dollars. Anything else for you today?"

Five dollars. I can do that. There is no shaking with the Prozac.

CHAPTER 43

Ball and Chain

THIS IS MY new daily routine: I wake up and take a pill. Before bed I take another pill.

Laiah comes into the bathroom while I'm putting the pill bottles in the mirrored medicine cabinet. "Aaron will see those bottles every time he reaches for his toothbrush."

I raise an eyebrow. "He knows I'm taking medicine."

"But you should never let him see the bottles. And never let him see you swallow a pill. You shouldn't do anything to remind him that you're broken."

The pill bottles go to the back of my closet shelf, behind my shoes. I can see Laiah's point. Aaron walks on eggshells around me. He never knows how a benign comment might be misconstrued. If he steps to the right, he might trigger an explosion. If he steps left, he might trigger a dam-breaking burst of tears. If he does nothing, there is no limit to the misinterpretation his silence could induce.

Morning and night I swallow my pills, but I don't know the prescription to fix my marriage. Dr. Amen says that the strength of a relationship is cemented by the brain's limbic system. As you grow close to someone in an intimate relationship like marriage, the trunk and branches of the brain's limbic system grow larger. You can measure the development of a relationship by physical changes in the brain. When an intimate relationship is damaged, it is physically painful, like cutting down a tree in your head. Wounded trees ooze sap. Wounded limbic systems bleed anger. This is why it's nearly impossible to have a civil divorce.

I don't want this to happen to Aaron and me. I love him and I know he loves me, but sometimes we look at each other and see strangers. He comes home from Goodyear one afternoon to find me curled in a ball in the middle of the living room floor, surrounded by boxes of unopened Christmas decorations. It can't be easy living in the same house as someone with depression. Danny's teacher told me she's worried because he plays alone at recess. Kate clings to me like a dryer sheet on flannel. Jack doesn't speak. He's seventeen months old and he won't look me in the eye or try to communicate. I'm worried he might be autistic. Tanner seems fine, but what if I've damaged something under the surface in him that will flare up in the future?

I try to be happy. I try to put on the smile, but it seems the medicine is taking forever to work. I once had a pen explode in my hand on the very day I'd chosen to wear my favorite white blouse. At the sink in the girls' restroom, the harder I scrubbed, the more the ink spread until the white porcelain was smeared with black, the air dryer had ink handprints, and the floor around the garbage was littered with wadded-up, black-stained paper towels. There was black ink on my pants, blouse, and on my history textbook. The rest of the day the ink spread to whatever or whomever I touched. Looking around my house, I see my black handprints on every surface, on the side of Kate's cheek and around the chub of Jack's little arm.

～♈～

WHILE AARON AND I were engaged, he joined my family for a Fourth of July camping trip. We weren't married, so I slept in the camp trailer while he stayed in a zipped-closed tent with my younger brother who had eaten chili beans on his roasted hot dog.

But that wasn't the bad part.

Instead of driving our reliable Ford diesel truck, my dad had decided to pull the camp trailer with his ancient blue farm truck. It had an old gas engine and was held together with scrap wire and welding. The rest of my family rode to the mountain with Mom in the comfort of the air-conditioned minivan, but Aaron—in a measure of goodwill and desire to become better acquainted with his soon-to-be father-in-law—volunteered to ride with Dad.

Forty minutes into the drive, the blue truck vapor locked. Vapor locking is something gas engines do—perhaps a combination of overheating and fuel flooding; I can't say for certain because I don't understand the mechanics. All I know is there was a *lot* of smoke, and the truck that was pulling all our food and my bed and bathroom for the weekend, wasn't moving.

By the time the rest of the family came back for us, Aaron was chained to the front of the truck, pulling with all his might while my dad pushed the back of the truck. Taking the steering wheel, my job was to keep the gears in neutral while attempting to master a dance combo step of tapping on and off the gas pedal and pumping with precise pressure at the opportune moment to get the engine rolling. *Tap, release, pump, tap, tap, release, pump.* When the engine didn't turn over, Dad appeared in the window, reaching across my lap, fiddling with the gearshift and barking repeat instructions about the tapping-pumping pattern. Through the windshield I could see Aaron bent over, panting to catch his breath, sweat pouring down his face. His shirt was plastered to his back and he kept hefting up the chain around his waist in the way a man hoists up loose pants without a belt. I can only hope we'd unhooked the camp trailer before Aaron started pulling.

The incident became one of our favorite family legends, retold and reenacted with fits of laughter—the legend of how Aaron proved what he would endure in order to marry me. Now I have become Aaron's ball and chain. I am the vapor locked, rusty old truck—the dead weight Aaron must pull.

He is chained to me. He's chained to our business. He's pulling the weight of the housework, the cooking, getting the kids ready for school. With our printing business, he's doing the work equivalent of three people. We can't go back and undo starting the magazine. We are stalled in the middle on our way to camp and we can't go back, but our engine is smoking, and we don't know how to move forward.

Aaron must be tired of towing the load.

———

DURING THIS TIME our family is saved by Grace.

Grace is a seven-week-old chocolate Labrador puppy. Her brown eyes are huge and dewy; we could all absolutely melt into the pupil pools beneath her puppy lashes. We are puppy-sitting for our friends Keith and Marsha. Animal therapy could not have arrived at a more opportune time. Grace works her magic and becomes a fuzzy cushion for our worn-out family. In her small furry body, she holds the love and affection we need right now.

Grace bounces out the backdoor, her little legs trying to keep up with the kids. They send her down the slide and take turns holding her on their laps while they teeter-totter. She takes it all in stride. While Danny and Kate are at school, I open the door to the garage playroom and find Tanner lying in the center of our giant bean bag with Grace snuggled against him. Her little head is draped over Tanner's outstretched arm while he strokes her fur with his other hand. Grace has found her comfortable spot, snuggled tightly into the nook of Tanner's heart.

Quietly I kneel next to the bean bag and rub Tanner's hair. "Would you like some lunch, Tanner?"

"Mom," Tanner speaks without moving an inch, careful not to wake his play-weary companion. "Puppies are my favorite persons."

I have never trained a dog, but I experiment with training little Grace. From the pantry, I get a few moist puppy treats. "Come here,

Grace." I hold a treat in front of her nose. She looks at me with her dark eyes, eager to be obedient. "Sit." Grace drops onto her tail. From the corner of my eye, I see Jack copying Grace's actions. He falls to his bum and lifts his chin, hoping for a tasty surprise. "No dog food for you, mister. Let's see what I have." I rummage through the treat dish on top of the fridge and find a few Hershey kisses. Jack stands, stretching on his tiptoes, hanging out his tongue and yipping for a treat. "First you have to do a trick." I unwrap the candy and hold it in front of Jack's nose. "Sit," I command. He drops to all fours and pants like a puppy. I give him the chocolate and pat his head. "Good dog," I say. Jack barks. Maybe he isn't autistic.

At dinner Jack shows off his new trick to the family. Danny and Kate laugh in delight. Aaron smiles. Tanner climbs off his chair, unwraps a candy, and is thrilled to discover that Jack will sit on his command as well. We laugh as our three-year-old puppy trainer and seventeen-month-old human puppy interact. Danny shows us a poem he wrote in school along with his crayon-colored drawing of a heart:

Pets stay close
Right from the start,
Take them home and
Put them in your heart.

Grace bounces, wanting more treats. "Come here, fuzz ball." Aaron picks up Grace and holds her to his chest, stroking her head. "You are a silly puppy." I look around my kitchen and see a smile on every person's face, including mine.

—⚬⚬⚬—

JUST WHEN WE'RE certain we can't do another print deadline, Bob comes over to meet with Aaron and me regarding "news" about the magazine. Sitting at the kitchen table, I brace myself for the worst. I'm crouched, ready, and watching for the next obstacle to appear—like the TV show *Wipeout*—hoping I'll be able to dodge the sweeping arm, but prepared for my feet to be knocked off the platform.

Bob sets both hands on the table and clears his throat. "My colleague in Albuquerque has been pestering me for years to sell him my publications." Bob leans forward. "Now that you two have gotten a Southwest Valley edition up and going, he's even more interested. He's made an offer. I wanted to show you the numbers and see if you might be interested in selling."

The numbers add up to more than a generous offer—the best Christmas gift we've ever received. Aaron and I look at each other with a collective sigh of relief. We take the offer. His load looks remarkably lighter.

Bob leaves and I fill my hand with puppy food and head to the garage, calling out Grace's name. "Here puppy. Here Grace." She scampers to me, stops and sits. Her wet tongue licks up the treats from my palm. I bundle her to my chest and collapse into the bean bag, overwhelmed by the miracle of this purchase offer. I'm suspicious whether Bob really wants to retire as he claimed or if he is more aware of our situation than we knew. In either case, he has graciously opened an escape hatch out of our sinking ship. I bury my head into Grace's fur, wishing for a good cry, but these days I struggle to summon tears as much as I struggle to summon joy. The softness of her coat against my neck reassures me that one day I will be able to cry again.

AARON AND I decide to move to Utah. Without the magazine, we can live anywhere and we need help. We need to be closer to our parents. We need nature, mountains, shade trees, and seasons. Our kids need their grandparents.

Aaron sends out his resume and within two days he gets a phone call from a business in Utah that has acquired a printing company as part of a merger, but they have no idea how to run it. They want Aaron to start yesterday, but they agree to wait until after Christmas. The job offer includes the opportunity to buy ownership in the company with substantial return on investment. We decide the new company is a perfect place to invest the income from selling the magazine.

I will stay in Arizona with the kids so Danny and Kate can finish their school year. Aaron will begin his new job, living with his parents and sleeping once again in his old basement bedroom. After work hours he will explore housing options and fly back to Arizona to visit us every other weekend.

Everything seems to be falling into place.

CHAPTER 44

Body

BEFORE AARON LEAVES to start his new job in Utah, we spend Christmas Day at home together. It's my favorite Christmas to date. We stay in pajamas all day long. After opening presents, Kate brings me one of her new books. "Mom, will you read this to me?" I wrap my arms around her waist and pull her onto my lap. She's been having non-stop growth spurts for two years and no longer fits on my lap, but I don't care.

"There's a problem, Kate."

Her eyes fall.

"This isn't going to be enough books. Would you like to choose some more?"

Kate runs to the shelf and pulls down a stack of books. We snuggle under a blanket and are soon joined by Danny, Tanner, and Jack. Aaron starts a fire. We cuddle on the couch, finishing one book then reaching for the next one on the pile. The rest of the day we play with toys, do puzzles, eat snacks, and play round after round of Candy Land. Throughout the day, Laiah makes herself scarce. I want time to last forever.

The following day, December 26, Aaron loads his bags into the back seat of the Taurus. I wait at the car door holding his lunch, snacks, and audiobooks for the long drive alone, then wrap my arms around his neck and wish him good luck in his new job. The kids stand with me on the porch waving goodbye as he drives away.

"Bye, Dad. Merry Christmas and Happy New Year."

Once the car disappears around the corner, we turn and go back into the house.

"Well, guys, it's just you and me. What would you like to do?"

For the first time in a long time, I have no appointments, no meetings, no deadlines. There is no magazine, no piano lessons, no seminary, no school.

My day is wi-*ide* open.

This hasn't happened since we first moved to Arizona when Aaron began work at Clover Financial, leaving me home alone with Danny. At that time I was anxious for accomplishment, desperate to prove my worth as more than just a mom. Seven years later, I want nothing more than to be just a mom.

<hr />

WITH AARON OUT of town, dinner is nothing more than a rotation through sandwiches, cold cereal, or macaroni and cheese. Tonight, however, we are going to our favorite fast food pasta place, Fazoli's—home of the $1.99 kid's meal with all-you-can-eat breadsticks and slushy lemonade. But when we pull into the parking lot, we see a canvas sign hanging over the door: *Pardon our Dust—Closed for Renovation*. A collective moan rises from the backseat. No breadsticks tonight.

Back at home, pouring bowls of fruity swirls, I think how perfectly that sign describes my life, so perfect it could hang over my front door: *Renovation in Progress*.

The other night, following my new prayer of *teach me*, I opened my eyes and did something I'd *never* done before—I began to draw. Artistic ability escapes me. I don't sketch, doodle, or trace. So I couldn't have been more surprised than to see my hands spontaneously open a notebook and rough out a scenic message. The picture showed a stick figure (my hands hadn't miraculously acquired the ability to draw anything more complex) hiking up a mountain. Next to the mountain my hand drew a helicopter. From the pictorial I understood that Ms. Stick Figure had been hoping for a helicopter to carry her to the summit, until she realized that without the strength and perspective developed while hiking, the top would have no meaning and she would be no wiser for her journey.

This was the first visual answer I've received to a prayer. My first divine pictogram. The message was clear: I'm in for a long climb. I'd expected to swallow the pills and feel better, but God isn't going to send a helicopter to whisk me up and out of my problems; rather, I'm going to have to haul myself out exactly the same way I climbed myself in—one step at a time.

In my college human development course, we learned that the five dimensions of personal wellness are intellectual, emotional, physical, spiritual, and social. In other words, mind, heart, body, spirit, and relationships. Finally, more than two years after teaching seminary, it occurs to me that the theme of the New Testament is *healing*— and not just healing, but being made *whole*. The goal of holistic medicine is to treat all aspects of a person, not just the body. I am broken in all five areas. Being able to see and hear Laiah makes me cognizant of the work required to overhaul my automatic negative thought processes. My heart and emotions are confused. I struggle to feel spirit and inspiration.

And there's my marriage.

Aaron has moved back in with his parents in Utah and I'm not wearing a wedding ring. People at church started asking questions, so I put on my ring again only to have it fall down the garbage disposal. I fished it out and washed off the egg shells, but it's pointless to get it resized because I will eventually return to my normal weight.

Since Aaron moved, I've met no fewer than five women who are newly single, having divorced after twenty, twenty-five, thirty years of marriage. I can't help but wonder—if they were able to make it through twenty years of marriage, what changed so much they couldn't or didn't want to keep going? In the past, if thoughts of divorce ever crept up in my mind, I would quickly extinguish them. I never allowed myself to consider any other option than staying married, as if the act of questioning were an insult to my sacred union. Lately, when someone asks, "Are you and Aaron still married?" I ask myself, *Do I* want *to be married?*

The question sits in Aaron's empty seat at the dinner table and on the side of the driveway where his car isn't parked. It sits in his spot on the couch during the quiet hours between 8:30 p.m. until I decide to go to bed, alone. In bed I put my arm over the empty space where Aaron should be. I don't want nine years of married life, memories, and limbic bonding to be severed. I don't want to be single, and I don't want to start married life again with somebody else.

So I can't understand why, without Aaron here, I am happier than I've been in years. I don't know what to do with this question except let it hang around until I have an answer for it.

ALMOST EXACTLY ONE year ago was my appointment with Dr. Thorpe. At that time I was hoping for a mandatory hospital stay and a surgeon who would cut me open and remove all the bad— as simple as getting a helicopter ride to the top of the mountain. Instead, what is actually happening is that I've found myself smack in the middle of a rare pocket of time and space where I have few obligations except to work on my own recovery.

I don't even have to sell our house.

Two months before Jack was born—during that time when our life was a cyclone of chaos and the real estate market was going gangbusters—Aaron had the idea to sell our house to an investor and rent it back until we were ready to move. With the new baby we were outgrowing our space. The market was high, so not a good time to buy, but a great time to sell. Investors were eagerly picking up rental properties. Aaron found an investor who bought our house at peak market price and agreed to rent it back to us for two years. Our two-year rental contract ends in June.

This means there is no for sale sign in the front yard. I don't have to handle a volley of phone calls and agent showings. Rather than tailing Jack with glass cleaner and a rag, I can relax and leave his fingerprints on the front window. This is nothing short of a miracle. Instead of having to vigilantly keep my house to the pristine level of a model home, I can allow my house to be what I need it to be—my infirmary. For the next six months, my house will be my own intensive care unit and I will be my own doctor attending to multiple fractures in mind, heart, body, spirit, and relationships. The first treatment will address *body*. I call this *Renovation Phase One* and start by joining a gym.

—⟢⟢⟢—

Renovation Phase One: Body

IN CELEBRATION OF the New Year, my mailbox has been overflowing with fitness offers. The new gym close to my house is offering a free *Introduction to Basic Yoga* class.

"Yoga?" Laiah questions. "Isn't that for scrawny, bald monks in India?"

I've never done yoga before—at least, not on purpose—but it's free, so what's to lose? Deanne watches the kids and I open the classroom door expecting to find stretchy people twisted into awkward poses with their feet wrapped behind their necks like human pretzels. No part of my body is naturally flexible—I'm the tightly-strung rubber band in every sense of the meaning—so I'm skeptical that I'll be capable of doing yoga, let alone find any enjoyment in it.

The teacher is not a bronze-colored guru wearing a white sheath. Her name is Trina. She has short-cropped brown hair, tightly-toned abs, and muscular arms, calves, thighs, and shoulders. She stretches forward and her sports bra reveals two perky round breasts—silicone, I presume. She is amazingly fit, and I wonder if she ever leaves the gym.

Trina asks who in the class has done yoga before; only three people raise their hands. She tells us that she used to be a body builder, and stumbled upon yoga during a stressful and sad period of her life and has become its faithful disciple. For ninety minutes, Trina is going to teach us the core poses of yoga. "Spread your feet out on your mat," she explains.

We gather borrowed mats from a box. I remove my gym shoes and socks and stand in my bare feet. At any minute I expect her to launch us into a painful routine that I will dread coming back to do the next day. I will probably quit after three days.

"Think of each toe separately. Move around on your big toe, put your weight on it, rub it into the earth, feel it connect to the earth." Trina spends ten minutes getting us equally balanced on all four edges of our feet. "Each toe is so connected to the earth, that it alone could hold the weight of your body."

In ten minutes I give more attention to my toes than I have since I played with them as a baby. For the first time in my life, I feel *grounded*. Energy from the earth surges into my feet and moves up through my body. With the class successfully holding mountain pose, Trina demonstrates the most essential aspect of yoga—*breath*. Yoga breathing is achieved by inhaling and expelling air through the nose with a heavy, vibrating exhale that sounds like Darth Vader. After several deep breaths this way, I realize that I'm a shallow breather. Here, in this stance, with all ten toes extending out to the earth for strength, and my body bathed in oxygen, I am no longer the wispy leaf of a woman who might blow away with the slightest breeze. I am solid. I could stand here forever, with my hands at heart center, drawing the breath of life from the earth.

The other poses don't feel as invigorating as mountain pose. Downward dog has the blood draining to my head, my face plumping like a ripe tomato. Trina spots my posture and comes over to press the lump out of my back with her hands. She leads us through the warrior poses. I teeter and fall out of position, catch my balance, plant my feet, and extend my arms again. My muscles feel stretched, but they aren't screaming in pain. Instead of exhausted, I feel powerful.

After class I go immediately to the front desk to sign up for a membership with a daycare package. My membership perk includes six months of free, one-on-one personal training. I've never had a personal trainer before. This should be interesting.

On the way home, the world seems different. I vibrate with the undercurrents of energy that pulse between the ground, the trees, the geese flying overhead, and the rays of sun. I feel alive in a bigger sense, a part of creation, more than a speck on the planet rushing here and there to pay bills. I feel connected to a greater purpose that is unfolding all around me.

CHAPTER 45

Mind

Renovation Phase Two: Mind

DR. AMEN'S BOOK sits on my nightstand. Every night I read and make notes. During the day I pay attention to Laiah and the things she says. Now that I know about her, I realize she never shuts up. What I could use is some strong duck tape, I mean duct tape, to keep her quiet.

When Christmas break ends, Danny and Kate return to school and my new daily routine takes shape. In the morning my eyes open at the sound of Laiah's voice. "Wake up. Hurry. Today is going to be busy, busy, busy!" Standing at the foot of my bed like a drill sergeant armed with a clipboard, Laiah shouts, "No time to laze around in bed. Hustle, hustle, hustle."

Instead of taking her words at face value and dashing into my day, I pause and study her.

Inevitably that makes her fidget. "What are you doing?" she asks.

"I'm looking at you." She is stiff and miserable, and I feel sorry that I've made her this way. "Come sit here." I pat the bed next to me.

"What? You want me to...?"

"Come here, for just a second," I insist, then wait.

She huffs, tosses her clipboard onto the couch, and with ladylike movements, she lifts her nyloned legs daintily onto the bed where she crosses her ankles, high heels still on.

"Feel that," I say, drawing in a thick blanket of air. The inhalation rolls deep into my chest and gently cushions my heart in layers of comfort.

"What is that?" Laiah asks with curiosity.

"It's breath."

"Breath?"

"It's life. Energy. All around us. Isn't it amazing?"

At that moment the sun pours through the drapes and kisses my cheeks with its warm lips as if to say, *Good morning, dearest. How did you sleep?*

"Wow, I've never noticed it before." Laiah shifts, trying to relax against the pillow, then she bolts up. "You have so many things you have to do today!"

Inhale. Pause. *Exhale.*

"I have *two* things to do today: be a mom and get well." With that statement I climb out of bed, dress in sweats, slide my hair into a ponytail, and wake up Danny and Kate. At 7:40 a.m. we all load into the van—not hurried, not frenzied, not running late—and sing Josh Groban's "You Raise Me Up" all the way to school. After dropping off Danny and Kate to school, the rest of us go straight to the gym. Tanner and Jack run eagerly into the kids' gym where there are more toys and friends than two boys could possibly need to stay happy for hours.

I do a one-hour workout, mostly wandering around looking at the equipment, trying to figure out how to use it. It feels incredibly self-gratuitous. Tanner begs to stay longer. I promise him we will come again tomorrow. "We will come every day this week."

Back home Tanner, Jack, and I prop pillows on the couch and settle in to watch *Sesame Street*. With Tanner on one side and Jack on the other, I close my eyes. Laiah looks down from her perch on the half-wall. "You woke up two hours ago. You *cannot* go back to sleep. You shouldn't idle here watching children's television programming.

Wasting time with children like this is exactly what keeps you from accomplishing anything impressive with your life."

Oh, Laiah. Bless her heart.

"Come here." I gesture for Laiah to come down from her roost and join us. "Let me show you something." I teach her how to caress Jack's baby cheeks.

"I never knew baby skin was so soft," she says.

Next we rub Tanner's bare toes. Laiah laughs in delight as Tanner retracts his feet. His cheeks bunch into a smile and his blue-green eyes ignite like sparklers. His laugh is a hearty belly giggle.

"Do all women know about this?" Laiah asks in surprise.

For the first time, she is discovering the perks of this motherhood gig. They've been here the whole time, but up until now, motherhood had to be all about work and nothing about pleasure. How else could we prove to our husbands and to all those paid working women that our job at home was not so easy?

Once the Elmo song finishes, the boys and I go to the backyard where I spread a blanket on the grass and open a book while the boys play in the sand.

When my cell phone rings, Laiah tells me to say that I am cleaning or packing moving boxes.

Inhale. Exhale.

"Hey babe. We're great. We just finished watching Sesame Street and now I'm outside reading a book."

"Don't!" Laiah interjects. "He'll think you're wasting time…"

Inhale. Exhale. Aaron does not track how I use my time.

I put down the phone and resume my book only to be interrupted by Laiah tsking. "Tsk, tsk."

Inhale. Exhale.

"Look at Tanner." I motion for Laiah to look over to where Tanner is humming a tune as he swings on his stomach, kicking the sand to the rhythm of his made-up song. Kids are so entertaining. How is it possible that I ever felt under-stimulated in their remarkable presence?

"You've missed out on all this time watching them play," Laiah chastises. "You've been a negligent mother."

Laiah can swing pretty quickly herself. Bless her heart.

THERE ARE DIFFERENT terms for Laiah. Dr. Amen says that Laiah is my automatic brain. Others would say she is my ego. My church describes her as "natural man." Some might call her Shoulder Devil, Debbie-Downer, or a Glass-Half-Empty Pessimist. She is me and she isn't me, in the same way my reflection in the mirror is exactly me, but not me at all.

Here's what I'm discovering about Laiah. She loves playing the role of victim. She is fueled by high-intensity emotions such as anger, blame, or rage, so she abhors her new restricted diet of truth and optimism. She claims to be starving and begs me to bring home some high-fat drama. If I feed her, she gets bigger, louder, and more demanding. I can see how people get trapped by their own egos. Like Dr. Frankenstein, if I'm not careful, I could be destroyed by my own monster.

So what can I do with her?

Tapping the pen against my cheek, an idea comes to mind: *Thoughts are energy, and energy can neither be created nor destroyed, only changed. I cannot get rid of Laiah, but I can change her energy.*

I'm doing my best do replace Laiah's negative comments with statements of my own truth. At the gym, instead of counting numbers for repetitions, I recite positive words such as faith, love, strength, power, hope, beauty. These help keep Laiah calm, but I'm going to need something stronger and more satisfying to her appetite than a few warm-fuzzy words.

Aaron would tell you that I am quite skilled at changing my mind, but a creature like Laiah is not so easy to transform.

—◦◦◦—

I'M PUSHING JACK in the baby swing one afternoon when my cell phone rings. Usually Aaron waits until bedtime to call, so I wonder what's urgent.

"Did you watch *Oprah* yesterday?" he asks.

"Who is this?" I look at the caller ID.

"I'm serious," he reassures. "All the guys at work have been talking about it today."

All the *guys?*

"You have to watch. It's amazing."

"Tell me about it."

"I'm not going to spoil anything. You have to watch it."

"It's recorded on DVR."

"Skype me tonight after you finish it."

I hang up the phone and search the sky for the spaceship that kidnapped my husband and replaced him with an alien.

After the kids are in bed, I click through the DVR menu. The episode is about a documentary called *The Secret*. Every guest on the panel talks about how to change thoughts. I pause the recording and run for my notebook. From the first word, I am hooked, my hand flying, taking copious notes.

Most people inhabit a perspective that life is lack and limitation.

I do this! My life is meticulously calculated to ensure that I could never be accused of having it easy or having it all. It's like a personal quest to make sure everyone knows how much money and time I *don't* have. Other things I make sure not to have enough of include sleep, vacations, appreciation, new clothes, and thoughtful gifts from Aaron. My "lack" has been proudly worn on my chest as a badge of honor. "He who lacks the most will inherit the Kingdom of Heaven." ....I swear I've read that in the Bible.

The biggest takeaway from the episode is that I've at last learned the tool for retraining Laiah, and it's better than duct tape. The tool is: *gratitude.*

Gratitude is a state of mind, inhabiting a mental place of abundance, fullness, limitlessness.

This gratitude concept ignites a revolution in me. Gone are my days of being queen of Lack and Limitation Land. My bags are packed and I'm moving to the Kingdom of Abundance where good that comes my way doesn't mean I've robbed it from someone else. There is more than enough for all.

Thoughts are energy. Positive attracts positive. Negative attracts negative.

I create my life with my thoughts. My job is to retrain Laiah, and gratitude is my tool. Before I go to bed, I look at myself in the mirror and recite a phrase offered by one of Oprah's guests. "I am ready for more good than I have ever experienced, imagined, or realized, to come into my life."

"That sounds dorky," Laiah chimes in. "It sounds like that *Saturday Night Live* sketch with Jack Handy: 'I'm good enough, I'm smart enough, and by golly, people like me.'"

"Laiah, I am *grateful* you can remember a *Saturday Night Live* episode from that long ago. You have a terrific memory!" I jump onto my bed feeling jazzed up.

"It's still stupid," Laiah calls after me.

I fall asleep repeating, "I am ready for more good than I have ever experienced, imagined, or realized to come into my life." If I keep saying it, Laiah will eventually repeat it for me. That's what automatic brains are good for.

In the morning Laiah is there, per habit, with her whistle and her clipboard, but I notice she hasn't yet put on her shoes. Maybe she, too, is hoping for change. She reminds me of Grace, our ever-anxious puppy. As soon as I pat the bed, she jumps on and snuggles into the pillow.

We breathe.

She is catching on that I don't want her to go away. She also seems relieved that I no longer expect her to maintain a constant flow of negative diatribes. It had to be exhausting for her. These days I don't rush into my morning without conscious attention to my thoughts. First, I find presence, and Laiah waits for me to set the tone for our conversation.

"I am grateful for the sun." We tilt our heads, letting the morning light bathe our faces. "I am grateful for breath. I am grateful for life. I am grateful for legs that can move. I'm grateful for lungs that can take in air and send it throughout my body."

We stand in mountain pose facing the sunny window. "Laiah."

"Yes?"

"I am grateful for you."

CHAPTER 46

Heart

Renovation Phase Three: Heart

I WANT TO know how to heal my feelings. My emotions are so muddled. One day I was standing at the kitchen sink when a fog of sadness settled over me. This was strange because my mind, at that very moment, was thinking very happy thoughts. My brain chef had served up an order of sad soup for no reason.

Another book on my nightstand is about opening the heart. Interestingly enough, at yoga tonight Trina taught us camel pose, a posture designed to open the heart. Kneeling on my knees, I bent backward until I could rest my hands on my ankles. With my eyes looking heavenward, my rib cage was stretched wide open. It wasn't particularly comfortable. My natural inclination is to hunker through life, cowered forward, sheltering my heart. In camel pose, my heart is exposed.

Still, every morning before I open my eyes, I hear Laiah's whistle. "Get up, lazy!" She flips a page on her clipboard. "You have a million things you should do today: paint the baseboards, pack the garage, catch up your scrapbooks!"

Panic rises in my throat. I might hyperventilate at the extent of my to-do list. Then I remember, I have no to-do list. All I need is to focus on my heart.

"Come here," I say to Laiah, and pat the bed next to me. She shrugs and rolls her eyes.

I pat the bed again.

She plops down and I take a few breaths until she is breathing with me. "Tell me, Laiah, what do I really need today?"

"You should take the kids to the library, weed the flower bed, prune the bushes so Aaron doesn't have to when he comes home, you should…"

"I didn't ask what I *should* do, Laiah. I asked, 'What is the one needful thing?'"

Laiah thumps her shoe against the bed. "I don't know."

"I will tell you." I breathe in deeply and stretch into camel pose. "I need to feel God's love. The only thing I need is to open my heart."

And I do.

The author of the heart book has extended a challenge to have a meaningful encounter with another human being without doing anything out of the ordinary. No baking cookies or doing yard work for a neighbor. The challenge is merely to pay attention to the condition of my heart and to be available for what comes next.

So during this yoga class, where I am literally practicing opening my heart, I notice the man on the mat next to mine. He is deeply intent on his yoga practice and there is a profound energy that comes from him. I can't quite nail down what that energy is: sort of a longing, a lot of need, but not in a "needy" way. He is bulked up with muscle so I'm astonished by his flexibility. He is not a string-bean-skinny kind of yogi. He is drawing strength from everything around him, as if he relies on that strength with all his might to get him through. I also sense a depth of gratitude and understanding—the kind that comes only with a cost.

After *Savasana*, we sit cross-legged and reach one last time to the sky, bowing our heads and offering our *namaste* which means *the good in me salutes the good in you.* At this point in my prior life, I would have rolled up my mat, kept my head down, and left class without looking at or talking to anyone. But today I stop to pay attention to my heart, which has opened a crack. And in this slight opening is a desire to connect with this young man across from me. How to start?

"You are the most flexible man I have ever seen," I fumble. Nothing about that sentence sounded right, but he doesn't judge. His heart is open.

"I didn't used to be flexible at all, but I have been doing yoga for several years now."

"How did you get started?" I ask, genuinely interested to know.

"When I got back from my first tour in Iraq, I needed something to calm my mind."

A flow of energy surges between us as if a third person standing witness to our conversation has reached into our chests, grabbed the broken parts in each of us, and joined them together, hand in hand.

When I had Lasik eye surgery, there was a nurse in the room whose sole responsibility during the procedure was to hold my hand. At first I resisted, especially because this nurse was a man, and I thought it strange and probably inappropriate to hold hands with a man other than my husband. But, disliking drugs as I do, I had chosen not to take the valium they had offered. One click of that machine making cuts and the bright light burrowing down into my eyes, and I grabbed and held tight to his hand as if it were my life preserver. I was amazed at the warmth and comfort the hand of this stranger offered me. When the procedure was over, I thanked the doctor and the multiple staff that had helped with the surgery, but I felt particularly grateful for this nurse who had been there to hold my hand. His role that day hadn't required any specialized medical school training, but his presence had made an immense difference to me. I've never seen him again, that I know of—I wouldn't recognize his face—but sometimes I can still pull up that memory and draw strength from the feeling of his hand holding me steady through my fear.

The Iraq veteran and I do this for each other.

"I'm in college now, and I do yoga every day. It gets me through," he says.

"Thank you," I say, "for serving our country." I mean it with a depth of appreciation I didn't know I could feel for a stranger. But we aren't strangers. We are both here in class with Trina, fighting our demons, gaining help from our teacher and drawing strength from holding on to the hands extended around us.

ANOTHER EXPERIMENT IN heart opening happens midmorning, when a neighbor stops by unexpectedly. I haven't brushed my hair or my teeth, and the living rooms looks like the used toy section of a thrift store after an earthquake, but instead of talking to her with only my nose poking through a crack in my door, I open the door wide, and surprise myself by saying, "Would you like to come in? Do you have time to chat for a minute?"

We sit amid the evidence of my lack of housecleaning, but I do something else surprising. I don't apologize—not once—for the mess, for my appearance, or for Jack's saggy diaper. All I have to offer today is me, imperfect as I am. It's not much, but this woman who stopped by is welcome to it.

PART OF OPENING my heart is learning to pay attention to my needs. This is a new concept and I'm discovering that I have seldom taken time to ask, *What do I need?*

A neighbor woman from my home town visited a therapist who advised her to make a recording of the vacuum cleaner running so that on the mornings she couldn't get out of bed, she could play the recording at the front door and unexpected visitors wouldn't question why she didn't answer their knock. My mother said that if the woman would just get out of bed and actually vacuum and tidy her house, she would feel better. And I do agree with that—to an extent. I don't agree with women having to hide our needs behind the sound of a vacuum motor.

A big part of this renovation has been uncovering not only my needs, but also my wants. It reminds me of an archeological dig, "Oh, this is what I need? How long has it been buried here?" In the process I am discovering buried wants, brought to the light of day like lost treasures. Over these past months, I've had time to think about what I want—not what Laiah tells me I *should* want, but what *me* wants. Surprisingly, it has nothing to do with big city life, talk shows, television appearances, or my face plastered on rows of magazine racks.

For example, I want a cow. A real, live cow. I want the four-legged, rawhide-covered, milk-giving, horn-growing, Warner-brand-wearing animal. The kind that goes "Moo."

For so long I've tried to suppress my roots, afraid that people who found out I grew up on a farm in a rural town would perceive me as a backwoods, uneducated, stick of a hick. Now I'm noticing how my urban home of asphalt and stucco walls feels like a sensory-deprivation cell. A yearning for nature has boiled up in me to the point that I crave turning dirt with a shovel. What I would give to pound nails into a fence post here and there, or lift a bale of hay onto a trailer bed!

One night I pass out paper to the kids and let them draw what they would like our new house in Utah to be like. My picture—I'm drawing these days!—includes a large yard with room for a garden, fruit trees, raspberry bushes, and a little corner for a milk cow. Hard to believe, but I hunger to pull weeds. I want a simple house and yard with at least one section of unmanicured dirt. I want a place where kids can roam the neighborhood and explore their own curiosity without adult supervision. I want neighbors at least twenty-five feet away, but not separated by towering stucco walls. And I want trees. Climbing trees. Shade trees. I want to sit in camel pose in the shade of a tall oak tree and open my heart to the world.

CHAPTER 47

Connection

Renovation Phase Four: Marriage

MY OPEN HEART has been telling me to talk with a counselor.

Here's the problem: As leery as my mother was about chiropractors, there was another type of doctor she suspected even more—psychiatrists. When my mom was a college freshman in the early 1960s, a girl from her dormitory had gone to visit a local psychiatrist. After dark, she came running barefoot through the snow, howling with all her might like a wounded animal. The next day, whispered from ear to ear, the shocked coeds repeated that the man had "stolen her virtue." From my mother's story, I imagine psychiatrists lurking in a subculture of medicine, luring female patients to their couches in the dark of night.

And now I have an appointment with one.

Technically, the person I'm waiting to see is not a psychiatrist. He's a family counselor named Greg LeBarron, and the only reason I'm remotely open to meet with him is that I already know him. We were early-morning seminary instructors together. Like soldiers who have shared the same foxhole, there is a trust that forms between adults who arrive at a church building before sunrise, armed with jokes and object lessons, in the hopes that sleepy teenagers might one day, in a time of personal crisis, draw strength from one lesson they learned during youth seminary. If there is one person I believe

I can trust with the tangle of complication in my head, it is Greg LeBarron.

I'm sitting outside his office in my parked car mustering the courage to walk in. This scenario takes me back to a similar scene, almost exactly one year ago, when I sat in my car parked outside of Dr. Erdmann's office, questioning the sanity of seeing a homeopath, and worrying if the treatment would include bloodsucking leeches. Even though I ended up taking thyroid and antidepressant medication, I don't regret seeing Dr. Erdmann. I'm seeing positive results from his treatments. This spring my sinuses are clear for the first time in years, and I'm not choking on pounds of mucus and sneezing round the clock. He helped me to recover my sleep. When I think back and wonder where I would be if I had taken the medications right off, I realize that I would still be trying to plow through life like a Mack Truck, oblivious to my thoughts, ignorant of my heart, and oppressive to my body. It was through Dr. Erdmann that I discovered Dr. Amen's book and learned about Laiah and my automatic negative thoughts. Deciding not to take medication was the best *bad* decision I've ever made. One day I'd like to do more homeopathy.

But I still have a long way to climb and the next step is getting out of this car.

The waiting room feels peaceful, like the living room of a librarian's house. I fill out paperwork and a secretary takes me back to Greg's office. We shake hands over his desk. He asks about our baby, who is now more a toddler than an infant. "What brings you in?" he asks, casual as can be.

"I've lost trust in my feelings." I explain. "My emotions have been so mixed up that I don't know how to make decisions. It's hard to feel inspiration. I feel worthless. When I need Him most, why has God pulled away from me?"

To me my world is caving in, but Greg's calm demeanor makes my dramatic situation seem…normal. "God never withdraws from us, but He will not fuel unhealthy behavior." Greg leans forward and puts his arms on the desk. "Do you find that you are happier, more relaxed with Aaron out of town?"

His question is like a tornado that has lifted my house off its foundation, exposing the private life within. "How did you know?"

"You are codependent...on your husband and on God."

This is a shock—I think of myself as an independent woman.

"You project a God who rewards your good deeds and punishes your shortcomings. You think you have to earn love, but God can't give His love on *condition* of a particular good work, because His love is *unconditional*." Greg talks candidly, no attempt to break this to me gently. "If you're looking for God to give you a pat on the back for every good thing you do, He can't do it. God will not manipulate His children."

My heart is pounding harder than ever, but there is no fresh oxygen for it to deliver to my cells, because I have not taken a breath since Greg LeBarron said "codependent."

"You depend on Aaron to validate your worth. Do you find that you analyze his every word and action as a judgment of how he feels about you?"

"Yeesss." My voice gets higher.

"Then you use that analysis to determine how you should feel about yourself?" Greg continues with zero delicacy, but I'm not offended, I'm swirling. I'm in a washing machine of all the many interactions I've had with Aaron—and with God—yearning for their approval. I need to swallow, but it's hard to swallow while you are holding your breath.

Greg looks into my eyes. "There is nothing we can *do* to earn love. We are human *be*-ings, not human *do*-ings."

That is so hard for me to accept.

For me, a prize must be earned fair and square. People should be self-reliant and work hard to earn their keep. Nobody owes me anything. My paradigm doesn't include free handouts.

Is this why I feel relieved with Aaron out of town, because I don't have to work to earn his love? With him gone, I can relax, let my hair down, and be *me* without feeling guilty for not doing enough to deserve him.

After the appointment, I add another negative repeating thought to my notebook: ANT #9 *Love must be earned. I must reject love that I don't deserve.*

—◦◦◦—

WITH AARON MILES away, I'm gaining a new perspective on my life and on our marriage. Up until now, I've been too close to my marriage to be able to see how all the little details fit into the big picture—a "can't see the forest for the trees" kind of scenario. This space of both time and distance is like getting an overhead, panoramic view, allowing me to examine the whole scene of my marriage at once, and I'm unearthing a few things.

First, I'm not a businessperson like Aaron. I'm not a natural entrepreneur like he is. I don't get a dozen ideas a day for awesome startups. I like science, books, and time alone to myself. I don't like to speed through life in a sprint, I like to take my time. I like being a mom and I want being a mom to be enough. I want to be able to be a mother without feeling that I need to run three businesses on the side in order to be successful.

Second, I want a healthy, happy marriage, where both of us can thrive in our individual interests. I want us to be able to reach up from our broken parts and hold hands for strength without getting all tangled up and tied down by each other's demons.

Third, I want Aaron to be able to be himself. He should be free to show his love for me in *his* way, not in the way I dictate. And vice versa. I want to pour love over Aaron with carefree abandon, like no-calorie gravy.

Fourth, I want Aaron to come with me to talk to Greg LeBarron. Going through my own harrowing healing process, I have wounded Aaron—deeply—and I don't know how to repair the damage. My skewed thinking and years of emotional roller-coastering have broken our marriage, and I need help to fix it.

How does a woman go about inviting her husband to visit a counselor without insinuating that we need "marriage counseling"? I schedule my next appointment late on a Friday afternoon, when Aaron will be home. "Will you come with me, for moral support?" I ask him. "Like you did at Dr. Thorpe's office."

—◦⁄◦⁄◦—

THE SECRETARY SHOWS Aaron and me to the office where we sit side by side in cushioned chairs and wait for Greg to enter. We don't speak out loud, but there is a silent conversation taking place in the air between us. By the way Aaron rubs the cuticle of his ring finger, I understand that he's known all along about my tactics and agreed to come anyway. I want to say out loud how grateful I am he's here, but he's studying the carpet pattern between his feet. In the nonverbal conversation, I hear his fear that Greg and I have concocted a theory, placing Aaron as the root cause of all my issues and have brought him here to "fix" the problem. He bites at his pale lip. His knee bounces with the helpless anxiousness of someone preparing to be skewered.

Nothing could be further from the truth. Unlike times past, today I have zero interest in placing blame or extracting coerced apologies. He doesn't know this yet, but more than anything, I want for Aaron and me to be able to relax and be content around each other. My arms want to reach out and encircle him with assurance, but my own skin is covered with nervous prickles. There's no telling what Greg will ask and how Aaron will answer. Aaron might say he doesn't want to be married to me anymore. At the thought, a solid lump rises in my throat and burning tears pool in the corner of my eyes. I'm crying before the meeting begins, which makes Aaron's knee bounce faster.

Greg strides in and hands me the box of tissues. Without pomp or pretense, he asks plainly, "What do you want from this meeting?"

Aaron defers to me to speak first.

"I feel a disconnect in our relationship. It's like a wall, or a lack of faith or trust in each other."

"Do you both feel this way?" Greg looks at Aaron. Maybe I should have clued Greg in on the whole "this is not marriage counseling" thing.

"I think we have injured each other," I say. "There is something off between us, but neither of us can quite put our finger on it. There's an underlying rift. Whether it's fear, suspicion, or just a lot of water under the bridge, I don't know, but I don't want a marriage that walks on eggshells."

Neither Greg nor Aaron say anything, so I continue talking.

"Aaron is gun-shy around me and it's understandable. Over the years he's never known what mood I'll be in when he gets home. He has to choose his words, his actions, and his gifts carefully, and even then, most of the time they trigger the opposite reaction from what he was hoping for."

The words keep pouring out.

"I want us to be emotionally close without being affected by each other's emotions. I want Aaron to be able to have a bad day without worrying that it will bring me down. And I want to be able to have a bad day without Aaron believing it's his fault and that he's the cause of all my misery. I want us to be able to weather one or two bad days without being convinced that either the world, or our marriage, or both, are coming to an end. I want truth in marriage—whole, complete, honesty. I want to be able to be myself and be okay with that."

After this massive word-dump, I wonder if I'm not as low maintenance as I used to believe. Do I sound too demanding? Is this too idealistic? Do I live in a world where the image of the gray-haired grandpa bringing daisies to his wrinkled wife is as outdated as the Polaroid camera? In this age of digital photography, do we Photoshop over everything so it looks good on the outside?

I'm tired of trying to always look good on the outside. The competing, the chalkboard, the scorekeeping—they're old. I'm tired of trying to be my husband. Can we simply live together and be happy without having to prove ourselves?

The three of us stare at the desk, which is covered by everything I've just said, and I begin to wish I hadn't laid so much out on the table. Then Aaron sits up. His leg stops bouncing, he squares his shoulders. He is fully engaged. There is no finger twitching or nail picking when he says, with solid hands, "I want all that, too."

———⟨⟨∅⟩⟩———

AARON FLIES BACK to Utah and we talk every evening via Skype. These computer interactions are more meaningful than many we've had in person, because in order to Skype, I have to stay in the office chair. I can't be cleaning, dressing the kids, or getting ready for bed while Aaron is talking to me. We are each other's captive audience.

He Skypes from the basement of his parents' house and we talk like we did when we were dating, only back then we were both using wall telephones with thirty-foot-long cords. The conversations are low pressure and, much like the time while we were engaged to be married, our plans revolve around when we can see each other again and finding a place to live together once June comes.

He asks about yoga. I ask about his new job. We get reacquainted. He asks, "What did you learn from Greg today?"

"I learned that conflict in marriage is healthy."

"That's a relief."

"It's actually not good to be like those couples in church who stand up and say they have never fought a day in their life. That means one of them has completely dissolved into the other person."

"Interesting," Aaron says.

"Healthy conflict is necessary for growth." I explain how the resolution of conflict increases intimacy—not just sex (although this is the reason why make-up sex is so good)—but emotional intimacy, intellectual intimacy, spiritual intimacy, even social intimacy. Greg had pointed out that people with brains and opinions tend to be more interesting to be around. "So conflict is okay as long as it leads down a road toward mutual resolution. What you have to watch out for is contention. Contention is not okay, especially when it's based in anger, which destroys communication."

"How do you keep from getting angry?" Aaron asks.

"I thought this was really interesting. Greg said that all anger stems from fear, so when one person gets angry, you have to go to the root of the issue—what is the fear? Anger is a sign that something a person cares about, values, or needs is being threatened. So you have to step back, ignore the anger, and find the deeper meaning."

Greg has "assigned me" to be open with Aaron, to share the processes I'm working through. It helps. Of course, there are the homework assignments that feel entirely phony, like practicing communicating through statements of "I care, I need, I value." But over time, those phrases feel less fake and more natural, and I start to like when Aaron talks to me that way. It's kind of sexy.

CHAPTER 48

Spirit

Renovation Phase Five: Spirit

GREG LEBARRON HAS given me a homework assignment. He wants me to receive a letter from God.

"Don't you mean write a letter *to* God?" I had corrected him at our appointment.

"No. I said it right."

"How does one go about receiving a letter from God?"

"Take a blank piece of paper," Greg instructed. "On the top write *Dear Maleah* or however you think that God would address you. Then listen and write down what you hear." He wants me to report back when I've finished.

Back home, I realize there are so many questions I should have asked: How long did the letter need to be? Did he want it typed and double-spaced? What if God didn't answer by the next appointment, or what if He didn't have anything special to say to me?

After the kids are asleep, I kneel by my bed with a blank page in my notebook. Laiah sits above me. "God doesn't hand out His wisdom to any old nobody who simply falls to her knees and begs," she says. "You have to *do* something big to deserve a big answer, like climb Mt. Sinai before sunrise, fast for forty days, or read the Old Testament in Hebrew."

Believing that Laiah is right, I get off my knees. I shouldn't even bother asking until I've demonstrated extreme sacrifice.

I HAVE SEVERAL more appointments with Greg, but haven't received my letter. "I'm still praying about it," I assure him.

I believe in prayer and I know God has answered my prayers in the past. It's just that, usually, these answers come in roundabout ways, like through a scripture, friend, or nudge. Up until now, I've viewed my relationship with God like a game of twenty questions where I can ask things, but only in a form that allows for *yes* or *no* answers. *Should I take this class? Should I go to this college? Should I quit this job? Should I marry this guy? Should we buy this car? Should we have a baby?* The answers usually come in the form of warmth and peace that means *yes*, or a cold emptiness that means *no*. I've never considered that God would speak to me in words, using real vocabulary that could be written down, subject, verb, predicate.

My relationship with God has also revolved around noticing where He has appeared in my life, like a maid that cleans your hotel room while you are out. You never see the maid, just the results of the maid's work. That is how God feels to me—like I am a big beneficiary of His work, but I can't say that I have encountered Him personally. I've allowed Him to guide my steps, to gently point me in one direction or another, but I've never asked Him to speak written words to me.

—⁓⁓—

IT'S A HAPPY day when Aaron calls with news that he's found our house in Utah. I was getting worried we would be pitching a tent up Provo Canyon.

"How do you know it's our house?" I ask.

"It's feels like our house," he answers. "The backyard has a big garden area which is pretty full of weeds right now, but the soil is rich. There are no houses behind, only a huge field with sheep and horses and a big dirt pile."

"Any cows?"

"I didn't see any cows, but there is a llama. And you'll love this…" Aaron's voice is giddy. He sounds like the wide-eyed dreamer I married. "The street is lined with trees."

I'll take a llama.

Maybe this is the answer to my letter. My life seems virtually plastered with sticky notes from God who has been doing a lot of organizing and ordering in my hotel room.

Tonight I kneel down again with my pen and notebook ready. Greg says I don't have to prove myself to earn God's love, but right now I feel ashamed and unworthy. I'm ashamed of my depression and of the times I hid in my closet, left the house in the middle of the night, or exploded in Aaron's face. God has to be embarrassed by me, especially when so many women live in grass huts and don't have enough food to keep their children alive.

There's a scripture that talks about waxing strong in confidence in the presence of God. I yearn for that confidence, not to be arrogant, but to have a healthy relationship with the Divine. Would it be possible, one day, to see the face of God? Could I feel confident enough to look directly into God's eyes, so deeply that I could see into the soul of the Universe?

Maybe I'm not worthy, but I pray anyway.

Help me. Teach me.

I am ready for more good than I have ever experienced, imagined, or realized to come into my life.

—⁓—

WE MOVE IN June, on Jack's second birthday. Poor Jack, spending yet another birthday strapped down for a ten-hour voyage in the minivan.

A few weeks in our new house and there are healthy signs of life in the neglected strawberry patch I'm nurturing. It helped to pull the choke-weeds out. Plus, a little water and fertilizer can work wonders. We've made friends with the llama by feeding it treats and petting its nose over the backyard fence. The kids have named it Choco-Villain. Really, is there any explanation for how children choose pet names? The llama, though friendly, has a possessed demon look in its eyes. The summer nights here in Utah are cool and refreshing, but with Choco-Villain stationed through a thin barrier of flimsy chain link, I can't commit to sleep with our door open.

When I received my letter from God before moving, it didn't arrive in written form after all, but in a series of images, sort of a personalized home movie. I did my best to translate those images into words, which are recorded in my handwriting—in my notebook, of course!—along with pages and pages of other lessons and messages from the past two years. The translation isn't perfect, but it's enough.

Among other things, my letter from God revealed hidden treasures about mothering.

One of the rare curiosities of mothering—different from any other occupation—is that you don't have to boast an impressive resume in order to be a good mother. Children don't care if you graduated summa cum laude or had your picture on the front page of a newspaper. My kids don't care what I look like, how many ads I've sold, or if my name made any "lists." I'm their mom and all they want is *me*.

Laiah used to say—and I believed her—that I had given up my chance to be successful when I chose to become a mother. This had me convinced that I had lost myself, that I had literally given up my life for children. The opposite is true. Becoming a mother gave me my *real* life. Before children, I was a slave to accomplishment, a puppet tied by strings of accolades to a strange marionettist who controlled my every move by offering a false sense of worth with strings attached.

Mothering has stripped me down and built me new again. Without trophies, awards, report cards, or recognitions, the work of mothering is every bit the barren desert I traveled two years ago. I nearly died of suffocation, like a fish out of water, crawling through that desert, begging and pleading for one liquid drop of admiration.

The rare, buried treasure of mothering is that there are no strings attached.

There is no boss, no declaration of personal value in terms of numbers on a paycheck. In this way, becoming a mother is the most liberating, feminist thing I've ever done. As a mother, I am the lowliest employee and the CEO; I am my own boss and my own worker bee. I don't work for a paycheck, but I also don't work to build someone else's agenda. I never have to posture for a promotion.

As a mother I am the only company in the world who has truly produced a one hundred percent original product. No one else in the world has created a Jack, a Kate, a Danny, a Tanner.

The heart of mothering is creation.

I get stoked up thinking about it.

In fact, every corporation, every endeavor, every operation in the world exists to support *me* in my work. Without mothers, there is no purpose to the world. Without mothers and children there is no reason to form governments, build economies, establish trade agreements, report the news, study medicine, or train an army. All these things exist to support *my* posterity.

I am mother. Within me is contained life and the purpose of the earth.

I don't mean to sound conceited, but that feels like a lot of power. Why have I always felt so *small?*

Laiah told me being *just* a mother wasn't enough, but who said it before her? Laiah has no original thoughts; everything she says comes from somewhere.

Because she said it, doesn't make it true.

Eyes

INSIDE MY HOUSE on a treelined street with a struggling strawberry patch and a llama over the fence, I stand in front of my bathroom mirror.

"I am ready," I speak out loud summoning a voice with strong conviction, "for more good than I have ever experienced, imagined, or realized to come into my life."

I've said this many times before, but today something happens. Somewhere in my brain, directly behind my eyes, I sense a physical *click*. My vision resets and—for the first time ever—I am looking directly into both of my eyes...at the same time.

I'd never been aware that, until now, when I looked in the mirror, I either looked in only my right eye or my left eye. I couldn't focus on both. I stare at myself in amazement. I am thirty-three years old and have never before looked myself directly in both of my eyes.

I continue staring into the mirror, looking deep into the dark pupils that sit in the middle of my brown irises and it's like seeing myself for the first time.

Let thy confidence wax strong in the presence of God.

For months I've pondered this scripture, hanging on to the hope of one day having the opportunity to see God face to face and to be able to hold my head up, look right into the eyes of Deity and say, "Thanks. For everything."

I never anticipated this development, to look at myself and see the Divine in my own eyes.

"Thanks. For everything," I say to myself and to that part of God that is in me.

Laiah sits on the bathroom counter, smiling. "Life is good," she says. And she means it.

All a mother needs in order to be successful is to allow herself to feel *loved*. And there is love in abundance to the soul with an open heart. We pause for a moment and bask in a swelling that is growing in our chest and moving up our body. *Fullness*.

"I wish Ms. Wickersham could see this," I tell Laiah.

"Could see what?"

"Could see what happened when an ambitious little girl grew up to become a *mother*."

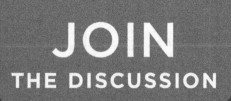
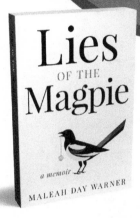
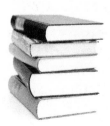

MORE FROM
MALEAH DAY WARNER

Download the next chapter

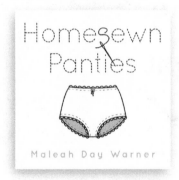

Follow the misadventures of growing up a Mormon Democrat in rural Utah. Maleah is coming of age and finding her place between Mormonism and Feminism all while wearing home-made clothes.

FREE audio or print download:

maleahwarner.com/homesewn-panties

Want the Latest News from Maleah?

Send us your email and we'll make sure you receive the latest news and updates about book releases, tours, classes and special offers.

Subscribe at maleahwarner.com

WANT TO ELEVATE YOUR LIFE TO THE NEXT LEVEL?

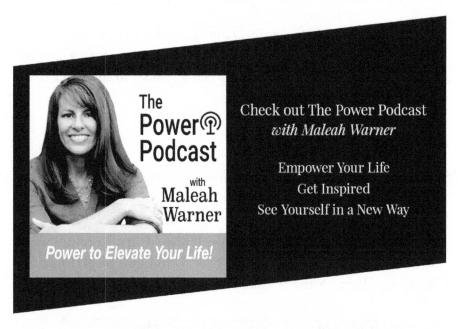

The
Power 🎙
Podcast
with
Maleah
Warner

Power to Elevate Your Life!

Check out The Power Podcast
with Maleah Warner

Empower Your Life
Get Inspired
See Yourself in a New Way

Don't Miss These Popular Episodes:

Ep. 12 The Power of Imbalance
Ep. 35 Side Door Approaches to Solving Problems
Ep. 39 What If You Don't Get Your Miracle
Ep. 55 Creating Energy

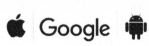

To receive The Power Podcast every Monday in your inbox,
SUBSCRIBE at maleahwarner.com/podcasts.

GRATITUDE

<u>To my family</u>:

Thank you to the real life Aaron, Danny, Kate, Tanner, and Jack. You've lived these experiences multiple times: once in real life, then again and again in the retelling. Thank you for being willing to share our story.

<u>To my Smashing Friends</u>:

It all began with you.
To Dave, the world's most smashing writing teacher. *What? Dave's not the teacher?*
To Caleb Warnock, thank you for being a *real* teacher.
To Cally Nielson, James Dalrymple, Janiel Miller, Loraine Scott, Maegan Langer, Melissa Richardson, Scott Livingston, Steph Lineback, Charmayne Warnock, thank you for reading parts or all of various drafts.

<u>Thanks to readers of early, middle, and late revisions</u>:

Allen Day, Angel Johnson, April Carson, Ariane Pierce, Bonnie Milligan, Daniece Crump, Gary Warner, Joyce Shumway, Justin Warner, Kathleen Wolfley, Kyle Crump, Lindsey Robrecht, Marianne Day, Mati Mayfield, Tami Day.

<u>Thanks to amazing editors</u>:

Renee Eli
Kim Clement: kimclementediting.com
Kristen Hamilton: kristencorrects.com

ABOUT THE AUTHOR

Maleah Day Warner is an advocate for mothering resources and education, particularly in the diagnosis and treatment of postpartum depression. She volunteers with Postpartum Support International Utah and The Emily Effect.

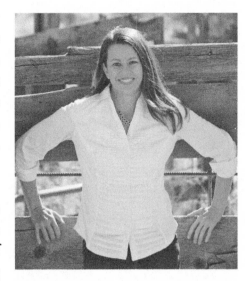

As a creative storyteller, she uses imagery and insight to capture the unseen magic of human experience. Her writing chronicles the otherwise mundane rituals of family life and turns monotony into a kaleidoscope of observations.

Also known as "MomMaleah" because of her passion for bolstering moms around the world, Maleah's goal is to educate, validate, and elevate the work of mothering. Her humor, warmth, and real-life examples make her relatable as she teaches local and online classes and speaks to women's groups to empower women with tools to heal heart, mind, and body. A healthy world begins with healthy mothers!

For more from Maleah:
Subscribe to *The Power Podcast with Maleah Warner*
Signup to receive her inspirational *Monday Messages* at:
    maleahwarner.com/subscribe.
Follow classes, speaking, and book tour information at:
    maleahwarner.com

Made in the USA
Las Vegas, NV
04 May 2021

22455871R00215